Clinical Short-Answer Questions
For Postgraduate Dentistry

Clinical Short-Answer Questions for Postgraduate Dentistry

by
St-John Crean
Zarina Shaikh
Liam Addy

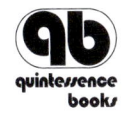

Quintessence Publishing Co. Ltd.
London, Berlin, Chicago, Paris, Milan, Barcelona, Istanbul, São Paulo,
Tokyo, New Delhi, Moscow, Prague, Warsaw

British Library Cataloguing-in Publication Data
Crean, St-John
  Clinical short answer questions for postgraduate dentistry
  1. Dentistry – Examinations, questions, etc.
  I. Title II. Shaikh, Zarina III. Addy, Liam
  617.6'0076

ISBN-10: 1850971021

quintessence books

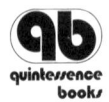

Copyright © 2007 Quintessence Publishing Co. Ltd., London

Quintessence Publishing Co. Ltd.
Quintessence House
Grafton Road
New Malden, Surrey KT3 3AB
United Kingdom
www.quintpub.co.uk

Printing: AZ Druck und Datentechnik, Kempten
Layout: Quintessence Publishing Co. Ltd., London

All rights reserved. This book or any part thereof may not be reproduced, stored in a retrieval system, or transmitted in any form or by any means, electronic, mechanical, photocopying, or otherwise, without the written permission of the publisher.

Printed in Germany
ISBN-10: 1-85097-102-1
ISBN-13: 978-1-85097-102-3

Preface

Preparing for postgraduate exams in dentistry requires an enormous degree of organisation and determination. Foremost is the challenge of maintaining a balance between preparing for exams and holding down a full-time clinical post. The pressures of work in dentistry and related specialties inevitably limit the amount of exam preparation time available to candidates wishing to pursue a postgraduate career. Traditional methods include self-study, attending revision courses – either after work, whole-day, weekends, week-long – and even signing up for distance-learning packages.

The authors of this text have wide experience in the provision of revision courses of all types through their work at the Royal College of Surgeons of England in London and have had the opportunity to talk to many of the candidates attending these events. It is clear that students are very keen to be given the opportunity to put their knowledge to the test before the exams, and they have repeatedly requested question-and-answer books to use alongside their revision texts.

To this end the Faculty of Dental Surgery at the Royal College of Surgeons of England has asked the authors to put together a series of patient-based cases and scenarios that reflect the clinical material beloved of postgraduate dental exams. The questions associated with each case have been designed to reflect the type of topics likely to present in a number of postgraduate exams, most notably the current MFDS and MFGDP diets. Each clinical case has been chosen from a pool of potential examination cases. The questions reflect the diversity of material that a single clinical case can generate. The answers provided to each of the questions in the text indicate to the candidates the breadth and depth of knowledge that will be expected for success in the exams. Where relevant, references have been provided for further reading. Not every topic will be covered, as this will require further texts, but the range is broad and detailed. Candidates will be expected to read the questions asked and answer each one before moving to the answers.

Preparation is the key to performance in examinations. The authors hope that this book will go some way towards providing a useful measure to candidates of how well their studies are progressing. If weaknesses are highlighted before the exam then the text will have achieved its aim. This will, it is to be hoped, encourage further preparation, thus reducing the risk of poor performance on the big day.

St-John Crean
Zarina Shaikh
Liam Addy

Acknowledgement

We would like to thank the Medical Illustration Department at the University of Wales College of Medicine, Dental School, for their kind help in reproducing the photographs, and the patients for giving consent to allow this information to be published. I am grateful to the clinicians and consultants who agreed to allow these cases to be used in this book, especially Mr Mike Fardy, consultant oral and maxillofacial surgeon, University of Wales College of Medicine, Department of Oral and Maxillofacial Surgery, Professor Martin Addy, Department of Restorative Dentistry, University of Bristol Dental School, Dr Margaret Hunter and Mr William McLaughlin of Cardiff University Dental School and Mr Nicholas Moran of Prince Charles Hospital, Merthyr Tydfil.

Authors

St-John Crean
Robert Bradshaw advisor in the Faculty of Dental Surgery,
Royal College of Surgeons of England,
Consultant in oral and maxillofacial surgery,
North Glamorgan NHS Trust
Cardiff University Dental School,
Department of Oral and Maxillofacial Surgery

Zarina Shaikh
Faculty education tutor, Royal College of Surgeons of England,
Final year medical student, Bristol University Medical School

Liam Addy
Specialist registrar in restorative dentistry,
Department of Adult Dental Health,
Cardiff University Dental School

Contents

Part I   1

Case 1	Wound healing	3
Case 2	Sore tongue	7
Case 3	Radiolucency of the mandible	9
Case 4	Mandibular radiolucency	12
Case 5	Parotid swelling	15
Case 6	Submandibular swelling	18
Case 7	Dental trauma	21
Case 8	Diabetic patient	25
Case 9	Recurrent oral ulcers	28
Case 10	Dental pain	31
Case 11	Lip lesion	33
Case 12	Toothache	35
Case 13	Dental pain	38
Case 14	Complications of unerupted teeth	41
Case 15	Facial trauma	44
Case 16	Sore gums	47
Case 17	Mandibular radiolucency	50
Case 18	Dental trauma	53
Case 19	Dental pain	55
Case 20	Xerostomia	58
Case 21	Retained roots	61
Case 22	Facial sinus	63
Case 23	Chance findings on an OPT	65

Case 24	Sore mouth	68
Case 25	White patch	71
Case 26	TMJ problems	74
Case 27	Facial pain	77
Case 28	Facial laceration	79
Case 29	Facial deformity	82
Case 30	Lump on the lip	85
Case 31	Mandibular radiolucency	88
Case 32	Dental pain	91
Case 33	Radiographic radio-opacity	93
Case 34	Lump on tongue	95
Case 35	Facial trauma	97
Case 36	Oral ulcers	100
Case 37	Oral cancer treatment	102

Part II   105

Question 1	Implant options in the edentulous patient	107
Question 2	Resin-retained bridgework	109
Question 3	Implant aesthetics	111
Question 4	Laminate veneer preparations	113
Question 5	Management of the discoloured tooth	115
Question 6	Non-vital bleaching	117
Question 7	Gingival recession and periodontal splints	119
Question 8	Management of palatal toothwear	121

Question 9	Management of gingival recession	123
Question 10	Partial dentures and free end saddles	125
Question 11	Management of the perio-endo lesion	127
Question 12	Tooth discolouration	129
Question 13	Edentulous ridges	131
Question 14	Gingival enlargement	133
Question 15	Fibre posts	135
Question 16	Painful gums	137
Question 17	Fluorosis	139
Question 18	Crown preparations	141
Question 19	Complex denture cases	143
Question 20	Root-canal treatment	145
Question 21	Infective endocarditis and restorative dentistry	147
Question 22	Designing dentures	149
Question 23	Toothwear and dentures	151
Question 24	Toothwear and composites	153
Question 25	Dentine bonding	155

| References | 159 |
| Index | 165 |

PART I

Case explanations

Part one presents a selection of cases that demonstrate the variable directions that clinical cases can proceed in an examination. The main topics covered include medicine, pathology, oral medicine, oral surgery and general dentistry. Where possible, references have been provided to support the text and give some pointers for further reading.

Case 1 Wound healing

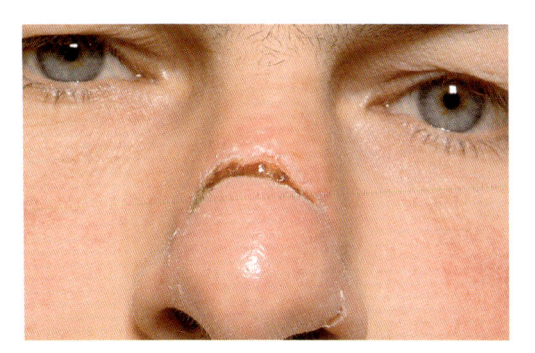

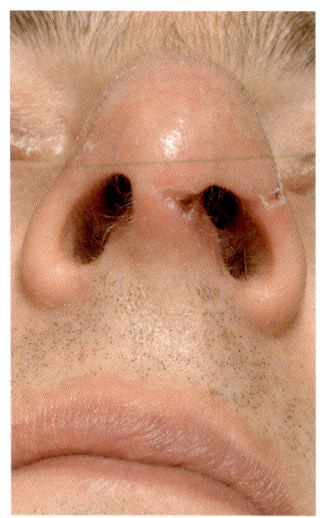

This patient sustained a human bite to the face. There is a circular laceration to the dorsum of the nose extending to the columella, and signs of dehiscence on the dorsum with marked reddening suggesting acute inflammation. The nasal tip appears to be vital.

Question 1:
What are the principles governing the initial management of bite wounds?

Question 2:
What are the stages of healing involved in a sutured laceration?

Question 3:
What are potential reasons for poor wound healing?

Explanation 1:
All bite injuries are likely to be heavily contaminated with potentially pathogenic bacteria. The management should therefore include the following actions:
- Take a thorough medical history.
- If patient compliance is poor, the wound very complicated and possibly requiring lengthy surgery, consider a general anaesthetic.
- Ascertain the patient's current tetanus status.
- Anaesthetise the wound with local anaesthetic that does not contain adrenaline. The tip of the nose receives an end arterial supply that will constrict in the presence of adrenaline, which, due to the length of time of its vasoconstrictor action, may result in tissue ischaemia.
- Thoroughly irrigate and scrub the wound with an antibacterial agent. The last solution to be used on the wound before suturing should always be saline.
- Suture the laceration using 4/0 resorbable, undyed sutures (for instance, Vicryl), for deep layers and 5/0 or 6/0 non-resorbable, monofilament sutures (for instance, nylon) for the skin layer.
- Prescribe high-dose oral broad-spectrum antibiotics and a topical antibiotic ointment.
- Review after one week for removal of sutures.
- Give clear instructions on scar management – for instance, massage and avoiding direct sunlight for the first three months.

Explanation 2:
In a sutured wound, the edges of the laceration are directly approximated, and therefore the type of healing that should occur is primary intention. There are three phases to this type of healing:[1]
- *Early lag/inflammatory phase* (nought to three days): Characterised by the cardinal signs of acute inflammation (rubor, calor, dolor, tumor, functio laesae), resulting in fibrinous adhesion of the edges.
- *Proliferative phase* (three days to three weeks): Increasing wound strength with the chemotaxis of fibroblasts, the formation of granulation tissue and type III collagen. Fibroblasts later become myofibroblasts and play a vital role in wound contraction.
- *Remodelling phase* (three weeks to one year): Extra cellular matrix stability increases with replacement of glycosaminoglycans and proteoglycans with chondroitin-4-sulphate. Loss of water between col-

lagen fibrils allows close apposition, reorientation and maturation of collagen fibres to type I collagen (Fig 1).

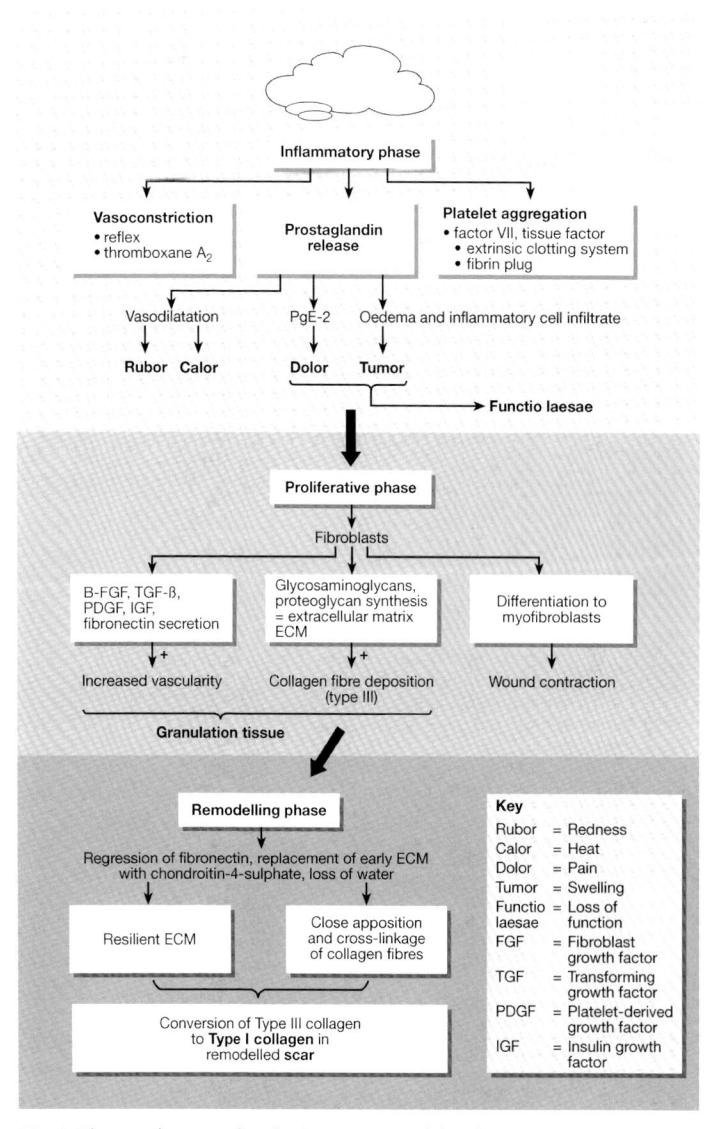

Fig 1 Three phases of soft tissue wound healing.

Explanation 3:

Local factors	Systemic factors
Tissue loss.	Age of patient.
Poor vascularity.	Nutritional deficiencies (vitamin C and K, protein, zinc).
Foreign bodies.	Poorly controlled diabetes mellitus.
Infection.	Malignancy with hyperproteinaemia.
Skin tension and oedema.	Chemotherapy or radiotherapy.
Poor wound care by patient.	Renal disease.
	Anaemia, Chronic hypoxic states.

Case 2 Sore tongue

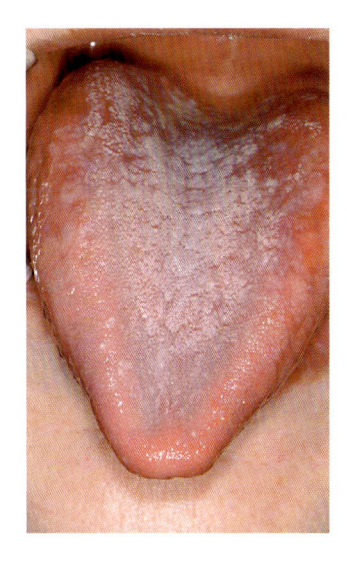

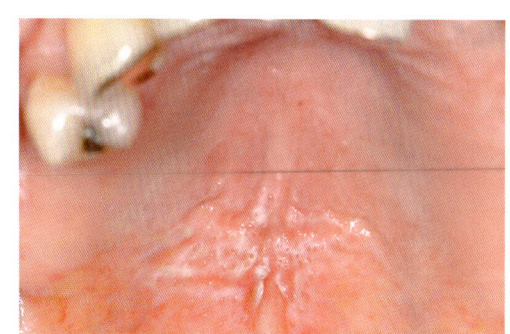

This 59-year-old woman presented with recurrent candidal infections, persistent sore mouth and swellings in the right and left parotid regions, which recurred whenever she ate, taking 24 hours to resolve. Her medical history revealed chronic joint pains, asthma, hayfever, insulin-dependent diabetes mellitus and depression. She is currently taking metformin and insulin, fluoxetine, propanolol, temazepam and becotide.

Question 1:
From the history and the photographs provided, give the most likely differential diagnosis that would explain this woman's sore mouth.

Question 2:
What further investigations would be helpful in this patient?

Question 3:
What is the relationship between diabetes mellitus and oral disease?

Explanation 1:
The photographs show multiple erosions/ulcers on the hard palate. There do not appear to be any visible bullae or striations. The tongue has a coated appearance suggestive of a high candidal load. From these features possible clinical differential diagnoses include: atrophic candidiasis, systemic lupus erythematosus or erosive lichen planus.

Explanation 2:
Recurrent candidiasis may reflect a haematological deficiency or immunosuppressive state, such as poorly controlled diabetes. Blood tests should therefore be carried out to investigate:
- Full blood count.
- Iron and ferritin.
- Vitamin B12 and serum folate.
- Random blood glucose.

The combination of erosions in the mouth, recurrent parotid swelling and joint pains are suggestive of secondary Sjögren's syndrome (not to mention several other autoimmune/immunological-based diseases). Haematological analysis should be carried out for the presence of:
- SS-A and SS-B antibodies.
- Antinuclear antibodies.
- Rheumatoid factor.
- Salivary duct antibodies.

In addition, swabs of the oral mucosa and an oral rinse should be performed for candidal assessment.

Explanation 3:
- Polyuria may result in dehydration and consequently xerostomia.
- Autonomic neuropathy may result in the development of sialosis.
- Glossitis and burning mouth are often seen in diabetics.
- Medication, such as sulphonylureas, may cause lichenoid reactions.
- Increased severity of periodontal disease.
- In poor control there is an increased incidence of candidoses.
- Surgery in poorly-controlled diabetics can result in impaired healing and infection is a common sequelae.[2]

Case 3 Radiolucency of the mandible

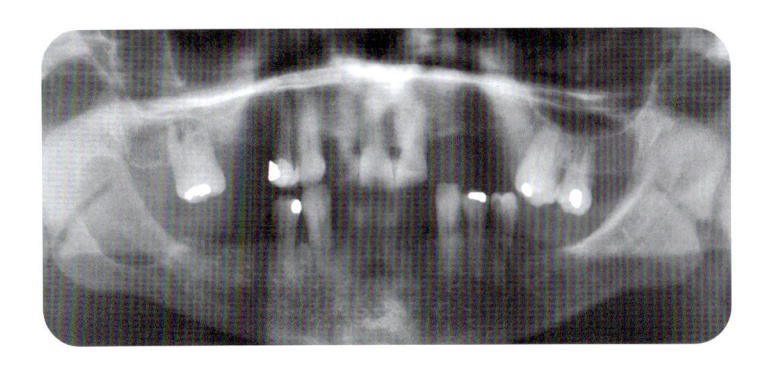

This 65-year-old man with a history of hypertension, arthritis and asthma presented with a three-month history of swelling to the right side of his face in the region of the angle of mandible. Orthopantomograph and postero-anterior X-rays of the mandible were taken.

Question 1:
What do these radiographs show?

Question 2:
What is the differential diagnosis?

Question 3:
What investigations would help you establish an accurate diagnosis?

Question 4:
Histopathological analysis gives a diagnosis of an odontogenic keratocyst. How would you manage the lesion from this point?

Question 5:
Are there any syndromes that the odontogenic keratocyst is associated with and, if so, what are the main features?

Explanation 1:
The OPT and PA mandible show a partially dentate mouth. The bone of mandible and maxilla appears to be of normal architecture. On the right angle of the mandible there is a large unilocular ovoid radiolucency with well-defined margins; it does not appear to have any calcific contents.

Explanation 2:
Although there are numerous causes of such radiolucencies, the commonest worthy of initial consideration are:
- Residual dentigerous cyst.
- Odontogenic keratocyst.
- Ameloblastoma.

Explanation 3:
Diagnosis can only be made accurately through biopsy and pathological analysis. Techniques that can be used to obtain a biopsy specimen are:
- Aspirate a sample of the contents of the lesion using a wide-bore needle:
  - Odontogenic keratocysts are filled with the insoluble protein keratin and desquamated squamous cells. The aspirate analysis will therefore show a reading of <4g/100 mL of soluble protein.
  - In contrast other cysts and cystic tumours have soluble protein levels of >5g/100 mL.
- Incisional biopsy of the lesion if the roof can be removed.
- Enucleation of cyst.

Explanation 4:
If this patient's hypertension and asthma are well controlled, the best management option would be to enucleate the cyst under general anaesthetic. Less commonly, larger and more complicated lesions may require marsupialisation. Because of the position and size of this lesion, the patient should be warned preoperatively about the risk of damage to the inferior alveolar nerve and mandibular fracture either during or after treatment. Advice should be given regarding a soft diet for six weeks following surgery to minimise the chances of pathological fracture. A postoperative radiograph should be taken before discharge, and the patient should be reviewed regularly over the next five years (annually) to ensure that there is no recurrence.[3–6]

Explanation 5:
Gorlin Goltz syndrome. Features include:
- Multiple odontogenic keratocysts of the jaws.
- Characteristic facies with parietal and frontal bossing and broad nasal root.
- Multiple naevoid basal cell carcinomas of the skin.
- Skeletal abnormalities – for instance, bifid ribs and vertebral abnormalities.
- Intracranial anomalies – for instance, calcification of the falx cerebri and unusually shaped sella turcica.
- Pitting of the palms of hands and soles of feet.

Case 4 Mandibular radiolucency

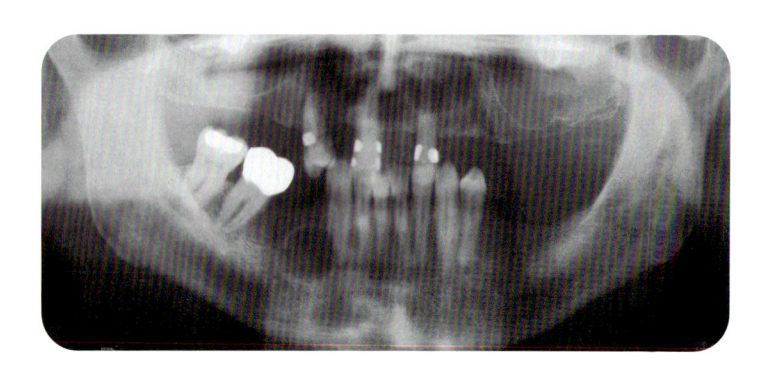

This medically fit 71-year-old man presented to his GDP for an initial check-up. He had no complaints. The patient was wearing well-fitting partial upper and lower dentures constructed by his previous dental surgeon two years earlier. An OPT was taken.

Question 1:
Describe what you see in the OPT.

Question 2:
Are there any tests that you might perform on clinical examination?

Question 3:
If the 43 is vital, what is your differential diagnosis?

Question 4:
What is the best way to manage this lesion?

Question 5:
What type of cysts can occur in the jaws?

Question 6:
What is the pathological basis of cystic expansion?

Part I – Case 4

Explanation 1:
The OPT shows a partially dentate mouth. The condylar heads do not appear to show any sign of degenerative disease. The teeth are heavily restored but there is no sign of gross active caries. There are some isolated flecks of calculus related to 47. The bone of the mandible and maxilla appears to be of normal architecture, although there is widespread alveolar bone loss suggestive of periodontal disease. There is a well-defined, corticated circular radiolucency in the right mental foramen region adjacent to the root of 43. It is difficult to see in this radiograph whether or not the lamina dura of 43 is intact, but there is no sign of decay or fracture in this tooth. There is no apical resorption.

Explanation 2:
Assessment of mental nerve function – remember this nerve supplies the ipsilateral lower lip and chin.
- Percussion of 43.
- Vitality testing of 43.

Explanation 3:
In the presence of vital tooth, the most likely diagnosis is that of a cyst. The two most likely types in this case would be:
- Periodontal cyst.
- Residual cyst.

Explanation 4:
Because of the size of the lesion it is advisable to perform a biopsy to ensure the lesion is cystic and to enucleate completely. Care should be taken to avoid unnecessary damage to the mental foramen.

Explanation 5:
- Odontogenic:
    - Developmental – dentigerous, eruption, odontogenic keratocysts, gingival, lateral periodontal.
    - Inflammatory – radicular, paradental.
- Non-odontogenic - nasopalatine duct cyst, nasolabial cyst.
- Neoplastic – cystic ameloblastomas, calcifying odontogenic.
- Pseudocysts – solitary bone cyst, aneurysmal bone cyst.[7]

Explanation 6:
- The contents of a cyst are usually hypertonic, and the cyst wall is permeable to water. There is therefore a net influx of water into the cavity along an osmotic gradient.
- The walls of cysts may also produce prostaglandins and collagenases that stimulate osteoclasts to resorb the bone surrounding the cyst.[8,9]
- The volume expansion in the cyst stretches the epithelial layer, inducing division of the cyst wall epithelial cells, thereby maintaining the integrity of the cystic capsule.[10]

Case 5 Parotid swelling

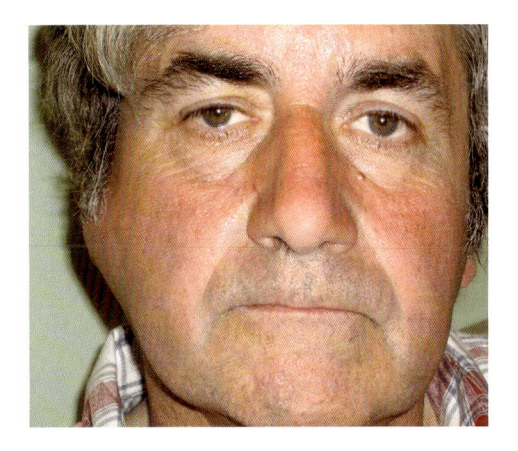

A 55-year-old man presented with a persistent, painless, increasing swelling of his right parotid gland. His medical history comprised ischaemic heart disease for which he had undergone a triple heart bypass and hypercholesterolaemia. His medication includes aspirin, lisinopril, atenolol and simvastatin.

Question 1:
Discuss what symptoms and signs you would look for on clinical examination.

Question 2:
Examination showed that the lesion was soft, painless and transilluminescent. There was no sign of facial nerve weakness, lymphadenopathy or saliva obstruction from the right parotid gland. It appeared to be directly related to the right parotid gland. What is the most likely diagnosis and how could you confirm this?

Question 3:
How would you manage this lesion in this particular patient?

Question 4:
What structures run through the parotid gland?

Question 5:
What are the two most common benign and malignant salivary gland tumours?

Explanation 1:

Symptoms	Signs
General malaise.	Weakness of cranial nerves V and VII.
Weight loss.	Signs of acute inflammation.
Night sweats.	Induration of the swelling.
Dry mouth.	Fixation of overlying/underlying structures.
Pain on palpation.	Regional/distant lymphadenopathy.
Pain on right side while eating.	Presence of a sinus/suppuration from parotid duct.
	Extension of lesion – for instance, intraorally (especially retrofaucally).
	Reduced/altered saliva flow from parotid duct.
	Tenderness to percussion of teeth on right side.

Explanation 2:
The above findings of a soft, transilluminescent lesion are suggestive of a parotid lipoma. Accurate diagnosis can be ascertained using an ultrasound scan with ultrasound-guided fine-needle aspiration and pathological examination or a T_2- weighted MRI.

Explanation 3:
Management must be centred around his complex medical history and the benign nature of the lesion. It would be advisable to just monitor the lesion and re-ultrasound it in view of its increasing size. Surgery should only be considered in this patient in the presence of any signifi-

cant morbidity related to the lesion, as the risks of surgery in relation to his medical history far outweigh the benefits of excision at present.

Explanation 4:
From superficial to deep:
- The facial nerve as superior and inferior divisions which give rise to temporal, zygomatic, buccal, marginal mandibular and cervical branches.
- The retromandibular vein.
- The external carotid artery.

Explanation 5:
- Benign:
  - Pleomorphic adenoma.
  - Warthin's tumour (adenolymphoma).

- Malignant:
  - Mucoepidermoid carcinoma.
  - Adenoid cystic carcinoma.[11]

Case 6 Submandibular swelling

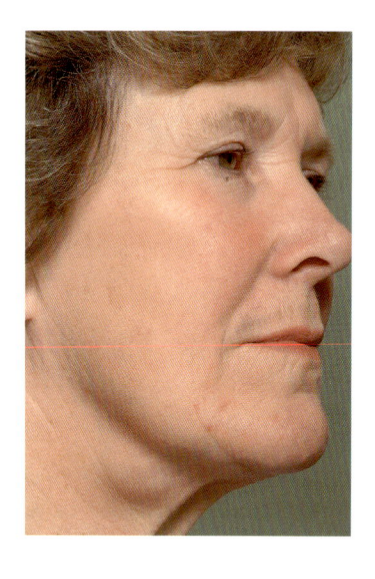

A 64-year-old woman with epilepsy presented with a five-year history of right-side submandibular swelling. There was no history of pain and the swelling did not alter during eating.

Question 1:
Describe what you see in the photograph.

Question 2:
How are you going to examine this lesion clinically, and what investigations may provide you with helpful information?

Question 3:
If the lesion is shown to be a pleomorphic adenoma, what are its characteristic histological features?

Question 4:
You decide to remove the affected submandibular gland. What structures will you pass through to reach the gland?

Question 5:
Which nerves could potentially be damaged by this surgery, and what would be the likely sequelae of their damage?

Part I – Case 6

Explanation 1:
There is a swelling of approximately 3cm diameter in the right submandibular region. There is no sign of an extraoral sinus and no features of acute inflammation.

Explanation 2:
- Palpate the lesion and regional lymphatics extraorally.
- Examine the lesion closer, using intraoral/extraoral bimanual palpation.
- Assess the flow of saliva from the right and left submandibular ducts, looking for evidence of mucus plugs/stones or suppuration.
- Carry out radiographic analysis using an OPT and true occlusal radiograph, a sialogram plus or minus an ultrasound scan and fine needle aspiration to ascertain whether or not there are any duct strictures, sialoliths or other pathology in the submandibular gland.

Explanation 3:
Pleomorphic adenoma is a benign salivary gland tumour mainly arising from epithelial and myoepithelial cells. It is called pleomorphic because it is composed of a disordered mass of varied tissues. It is an encapsulated tumour. The features often seen in this tumour are:
- Ducts.
- Sheets/strands of dark staining epithelial cells.
- Squamous metaplasia and foci of keratin.
- Fibrous and elastic tissue.
- Mixoid tissue.
- Cartilage.

Explanation 4:
From superficial to deep the main structures are:
- Skin.
- Superficial fascia.
- Platysma muscle.
- Superficial layer of deep cervical fascia.

Explanation 5:
- Marginal mandibular branch of the facial nerve (CN VII) – resulting in weakness of the ipsilateral platysma muscle and the musculature of the oral orifice.
- Lingual nerve (CN Viii/ chorda tympani CN VII) – resulting in loss of sensation and taste to the anterior 2/3 of the tongue.
- Hypoglossal nerve (CN XII) – resulting in loss of motor supply to the ipsilateral half of the tongue.

Case 7 Dental trauma

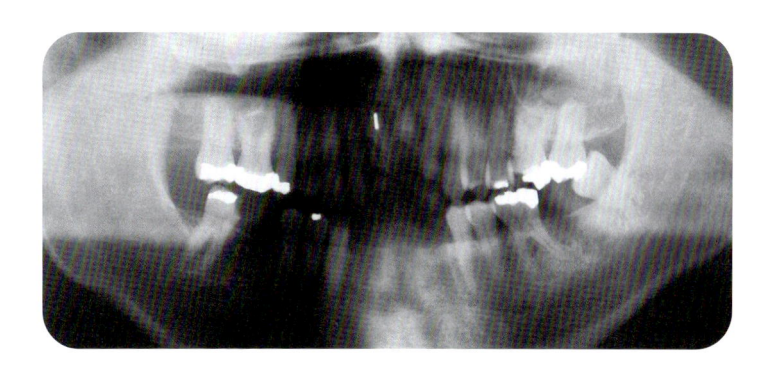

This 43-year-old man had sustained injuries to his face and mouth following a fall one week earlier. On examination, 11, 21, 22, 31, 32, 33 and 41 were avulsed or fractured and left at the site of injury and 26 and 47 had fractured cusps. The patient was extremely anxious about his appearance. Medically he was fit and well and not taking any medication.

Question 1:
He is historically a very irregular dental attender, but has come to you for treatment of the spaces at the front of his mouth. Using the OPT provided, what treatment sequence would you suggest for this patient?

Question 2:
He decides that he would like to have implants to replace his front teeth. What are the selection criteria for an implant patient?

Question 3:
What are the possible complications associated with implants?

Question 4:
What are the principles for ensuring that osseointegration of implants occurs?

Explanation 1:
- Carry out a thorough extraoral and intraoral examination to ascertain whether there are any signs of bony fractures. Assess the general health of the mouth, the presence of active dental disease and record the extent of injury to the dentition.
- In this case there is no sign of active decay or periodontal disease, so treatment of the fractured teeth can commence.
- Acquire study models, preferably mounted on a semi-adjustable articulator – for instance, a Dentatus articulator.
- Extract all fractured fragments of root remaining from 11, 12, 22.
- Restore all fractured cusps (36, 46) using either amalgam or composite restorations.
- Consider the options for restoration of the space anteriorly. These are dependent on complete assessment of the patient's general oral health and occlusion. Options include:
  - P/. acrylic denture, either spoon or Every design, with adjustments as bone remodels. Consider a lower partial acrylic denture.
  - Resin-retained bridges 12-11 and 23-22-21. The fact that the lower arch space crosses the midline and the adjacent teeth are all restoration and disease-free would make retention of a resin-retained bridge difficult and preparation for fixed movable bridgework very destructive. A lower denture or an implant-retained bridge would possibly be a better option in this arch.
  - Implants to retain bridgework across the upper and lower arch spaces anteriorly.

Explanation 2:
- A patient who is generally healthy and not suffering from uncontrolled systemic disease – for instance, diabetes mellitus. Extreme caution should be exercised when considering patients with bleeding disorders.
- A non-smoker.
- Good oral hygiene status.
- Patient cooperation.
- Favourable anatomy – adequate bone quality, depth and width, as well as adequate access.

Explanation 3:
Complications associated with implant surgery (or for that matter any surgical procedure) can be general or specific and can be:
- Immediate – during the operation or within the first 24 hours.
- Early – during the first week.
- Late – up to one month post-operative, or long-term.[12–14]

Immediate local complications of implant surgery include:
- Inadequate anaesthesia; damage to adjacent structures to the implant site – for instance, nerves, blood vessels, teeth, restorations, maxillary sinus; perforation of buccal alveolar bone; fracture of the mandible – for instance, in osteoporotic/atrophic cases; fracture of the implant, swallowing or aspiration of implant component.

Immediate general complications include:
- Complications related to type of anaesthetic used – for instance, allergic reaction to anaesthetic; bleeding disorders, respiratory and cardiac events in the case of a general anaesthetic.

Early local complications include:
- Swelling; numbness related to nerve damage; wound infection; cellulitis or abscess formation; wound dehiscence; osteitis; peri-implantitis.

Early general complications include:
- Haemorrhage; pain; septicaemia, respiratory complications of general anaesthetic – for instance, chest infection, deep vein thrombosis following a period of immobility in hospital bed.

Late local complications include:
- Loss of implant; bone loss or perforation into sinus/ inferior dental canal secondary to infection; prolonged anaesthesia/paraesthesia secondary to nerve damage; neuralgia secondary to nerve damage.

Long-term complications include:
- Permanent anaesthesia/paraesthesia associated with nerve damage; loss of adjacent bone+/- teeth secondary to chronic infection; loss of implant.

Explanation 4:
- Direct contact of implant with bone.
- Insert bone into a surgically prepared site using slow rotary drills of increasing size.
- Keep the temperature of the surgical site below 47°C to minimise damage to osteoblasts.
- The mucosa's health over or around the implant should be optimal.
- Ideally loading should occur only after osseointegration has occurred.[14]

Case 8 Diabetic patient

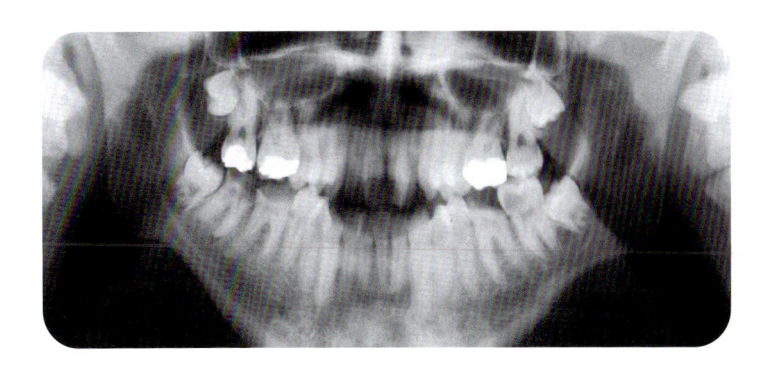

This 19-year-old complained of 'rotten teeth'. He had had no pain but was concerned about the state of his mouth. He has insulin-dependent diabetes.

Question 1:
Describe what you see in this OPT.

Question 2:
Discuss the treatment pathway that you would recommend to him.

Question 3:
What are the management principles when treating people with diabetes?

Question 4:
What types of diabetes mellitus exist?

Question 5:
What are the metabolic effects of a lack of insulin?

Explanation 1:
The OPT shows a fully dentate mouth. The bone levels are within normal limits throughout the mouth. There is a very high caries rate. From the OPT caries can be seen in 27, 37, 36, 46 and 47. It is not possible to assess radiographically the caries status of the anterior teeth in this OPT. There is periapical widening associated with 37 and 47.

Explanation 2:
The most important factor in the care of this patient is the management of infection, as insulin-dependent diabetes can be destabilised in the presence of infection. The treatment plan of choice for this patient would therefore be:
- Extraction of all unrestorable teeth with post-extraction antibiotics.
- Diet and oral hygiene counselling.
- Stabilisation of all restorable decayed teeth.
- Review of diet and oral hygiene after one month.
- Definitive restoration of all restorable teeth.
- Regular follow-up every six months.

Explanation 3:
- Treatment should be timed to avoid disturbing routine insulin administration or meals; give appointments first thing in morning and try not to keep the patient waiting too long.
- Use local anaesthesia/sedation for routine dentistry to minimise stress.
- In the UK, general anaesthesia should be carried out only under expert supervision in hospital (exception in Wales).
- Recognise any diabetic complications swiftly – for instance, hypoglycaemia, hyperglycaemia.

Explanation 4:
- Type I diabetes – insulin-dependent. Onset usually in young people. Caused by the destruction of pancreatic beta cells.
- Type II diabetes – non-insulin dependent. Patients have lost their sensitivity to insulin. Generally older age group.
- Gestational diabetes – Secondary to pregnancy.
- Secondary diabetes – Related to failure or removal of the pancreas.

Explanation 5:
- There is a combination of glucose under-utilisation and excessive glucose production. Because glucose in these patients cannot enter the tissues, it exerts an increased osmotic effect in filtered fluid in the kidney, resulting in a compensatory polyuria, which may lead to dehydration.
- There is a net breakdown of protein from muscle to make glucose. This use of protein stores reduces the availability of proteins for the production of immune cells and wound-healing components. The result is susceptibility to infection and poor wound healing, as well as breakdown and loss of muscle bulk.
- Insulin deficiency leads to lipolysis of triglycerides into free fatty acids which are then converted into acetyl-coenzyme A. Ketone bodies are produced in the production of energy via this pathway, and the result is the development of metabolic acidosis.[15]

Case 9 Recurrent oral ulcers

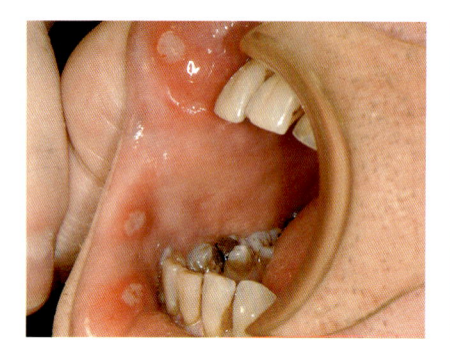

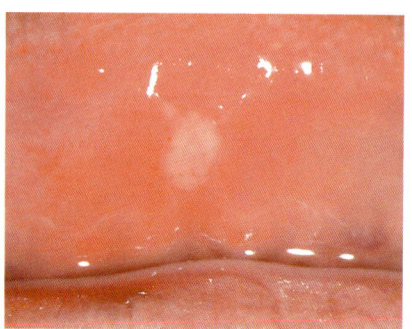

This patient complained of painful recurrent oral ulcers over the past four months. He had undergone a coronary heart bypass graft 10 years earlier. His prescribed medication was clopidogrel, atenolol, GTN spray, co-dydromol, fluticasone nasal spray, tamsulosin HCl, omeprazole, domperidone and pravastatin.

Question 1:
Describe what you see in the photographs.

Question 2:
Explain the clinical investigations you would perform on this man to ascertain a diagnosis.

Question 3:
What are the causes for recurrent aphthous ulcers of the mouth?

Question 4:
How can recurrent ulceration be managed?

Explanation 1:
The photographs show multiple intraoral ulcers on the buccal, labial and lingual mucosae. The ulcers are all approximately 3mm in diameter, with erythematous margins and a homogenous, non-granular base.

Explanation 2:
- Take a thorough history of the recurrence rate. Observe the pattern (minor/major/herpetiform) and distribution of ulcers in the patient's mouth. Take a family history.
- Take a thorough medical history. Check for a history of inflammatory bowel disease, diarrhoea, constipation, melena. Look for signs of Behçet's disease.
- Examine the mucosa for evidence of scarring. Look for clinical signs of other diseases that may present with ulceration – for instance, lichen planus/vesiculobullous disease.
- Carry out haematological investigations: FBC, haematinics (iron, ferritin, vitamin B12 and folate), ESR, autoimmune screen.
- Perform an oral rinse and swab for candidal assessment.

Explanation 3:
- Genetic factors/ family history.
- Trauma.
- Infections – may be related to cross-reactivity of bacterial and cell surface antigens.
- Immunological abnormalities – there is, however, little conclusive evidence to absolutely support any autoimmune/immune based pathology.
- Gastrointestinal disease – associated with deficiency of iron/folate/B12 due to malabsorption – for instance, Crohn's disease, tuberculosis and coeliac disease.
- Haematological deficiencies – principally B12 or folate. If pernicious anaemia is suspected, an autoantibody screen should also be carried out.
- Hormonal factors – in some women ulceration is associated with the luteal phase of the menstrual cycle due to the sudden fall in oestrogen levels.
- Stress.

Explanation 4:
- If an underlying medical cause is found – for instance, coeliac or Behcet's disease – refer the patient to a medical practitioner for treatment.
- Treat any haematological deficiency once the cause has been established.
- If no underlying systemic disease/deficiency is found, give symptomatic treatment:
    - Topical corticosteroids e.g. betamethasone or triamcinolone.
    - Tetracycline mouthwashes /antifungal medication.
    - Chlorhexidine gluconate (0.2%).
    - Zinc chloride solutions.
    - Topical salicylate preparations.
    - Systemic corticosteroids, azathioprine, cytotoxic drugs – only to be given under the guidance of a specialist.

Case 10 Dental pain

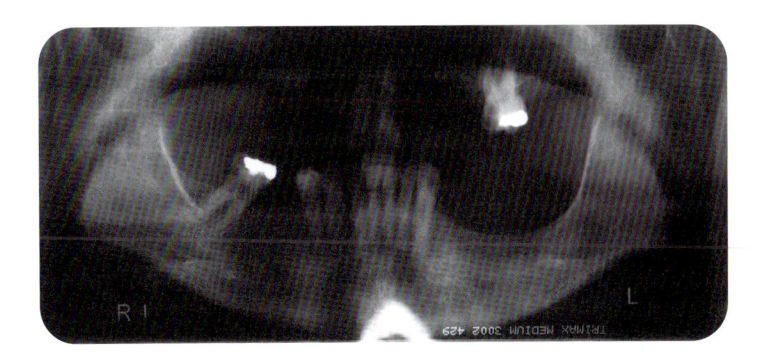

This 75-year-old woman complained of pain around her lower front teeth. She had a history of poor dental attendance. On examination, she was found to have poor oral hygiene and had been wearing poorly fitting upper and lower acrylic dentures for over 20 years. She has a history of angina, arthritis, hypertension, asthma, irregular heartbeat and an allergy to penicillin. She is taking salbutamol, verapamil, aspirin and glyceryl trinitrate.

Question 1:
The pain in her teeth is continuous and worse at night, disturbing her sleep. What investigations are you going to carry out?

Question 2:
What treatment do you think she will need?

Question 3:
How does fluoride work?

Question 4:
This patient has poor manual dexterity related to her arthritis, which is one of the main reasons for her poor oral hygiene state. What can be done to make oral care easier for this patient?

31

Explanation 1:
These symptoms are suggestive of an irreversible pulpitis. Diagnosis is achieved by:
- Examination of the dentition looking for caries, fracture and infection. All the teeth should be percussed and vitality-tested. A basic periodontal examination (BPE) should also be done.
- Radiographic assessment, either periapical radiographs or OPT.

Explanation 2:
The OPT shows extensive root caries affecting most of the dentition. The distal root caries cavity in the 33 is most likely to be the source of this patient's pain. Treatment may involve:
- Extraction of 33.
- Construct a new lower partial denture and make a full upper denture that will act as immediate replacement dentures following extraction of 47, 12, 11, 21, 26, which are all unrestorable.
- Restore all root caries affected teeth – 32, 31, 43 and 44 – with glass ionomer cement – for instance, Fugi IX.
- Give oral hygiene instruction and diet counselling and carry out thorough scaling of all remaining anterior teeth.
- Prescribe daily fluoride mouthwashes.
- Regular follow-up to reinforce oral hygiene and diet advice and adjust the dentures as bone remodelling occurs.

Explanation 3:
- It inhibits demineralisation and promotes remineralisation of early caries. It also affects the degree of remineralisation, thereby increasing the resistance of the enamel surface to subsequent attack.
- Fluoride, in increasing concentrations, inhibits the synthesis of extracellular polysaccharide.
- Fluoride is also believed to decrease acid production in plaque.

Explanation 4:
- Ensure that there are no difficult overhangs or plaque-retentive surfaces on the restorations in her mouth.
- Modify the toothbrush handle to make it easier to hold.
- Recommend use of an electric toothbrush with a small head.

Case 11 Lip lesion

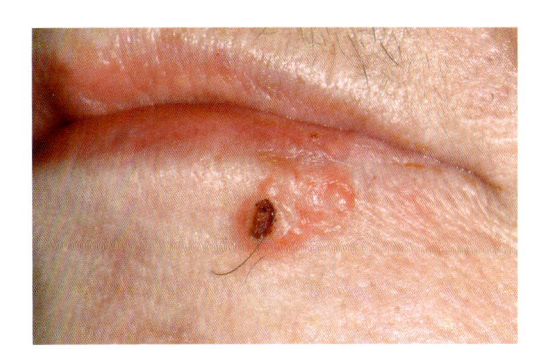

This 62-year-old woman was referred by her general medical practitioner regarding a sore lesion on her lower lip. It has been present for the past 12 years as a tiny freckle but has increased in size over the past three months. It often bleeds and leaves a scab. She is hypertensive, with a history of malignant melanoma on her back, which was removed six years ago. She is a non-smoker and very occasional alcohol consumer.

Question 1:
What is your differential diagnosis?

Question 2:
When examining a patient with a lesion such as this, what features in the history or clinical signs would make you suspicious of malignancy?

Question 3:
Would you carry out any further investigations on this patient?

Question 4:
If the lesion is diagnosed as a basal cell carcinoma, describe the appropriate treatment.

Question 5:
What are the histological features that would suggest malignancy?

33

Explanation 1:
The lesion is approximately 1cm in diameter. It is raised, slightly erythematous and nodular, with an area of scabbing. The above appearance, associated with a history of a freckle that has enlarged rapidly over a short period of time with a history of bleeding and pain, would lead to the possible differential diagnoses of basal cell carcinoma, squamous cell carcinoma, or malignant melanoma.

Explanation 2:
- The patient – tobacco-staining, high alcohol intake, family history, outdoor occupation, weight loss, cervical lymphadenopathy.
- Site – especially sun-exposed areas such as the lips or buccal mucosa in betel nut-chewing patients.
- Features of the lesion – persistent or rapidly growing lesion, ulceration with a granular/irregular base, induration, bleeding, irregular rolled margins, altered sensation, enlarged draining lymph mode.

Explanation 3:
An incisional biopsy performed under local anaesthetic is required to determine an accurate diagnosis. An elliptical incision is made at on edge of the lesion to ensure that the specimen contains a sample of both affected and apparently unaffected tissue. The sample is then sent in formol-saline for histopathological analysis.

Explanation 4:
Basal cell carcinoma does not possess metastatic potential. It can therefore be treated by a local wedge excision, ensuring that a good margin (4mm) of normal tissue is also taken. The defect can then be permanently closed.

Explanation 5:
- Drop-shaped rete ridges.
- Nuclear hyperchromatism.
- Nuclear pleomorphism and altered nuclear:cytoplasmic ratio.
- Excess mitotic activity and loss of polarity of cells.
- Deep cell keratinisation.
- Disordered or loss of differentiation.
- Invasion into underlying structures with penetration through the basement membrane.

Case 12 Toothache

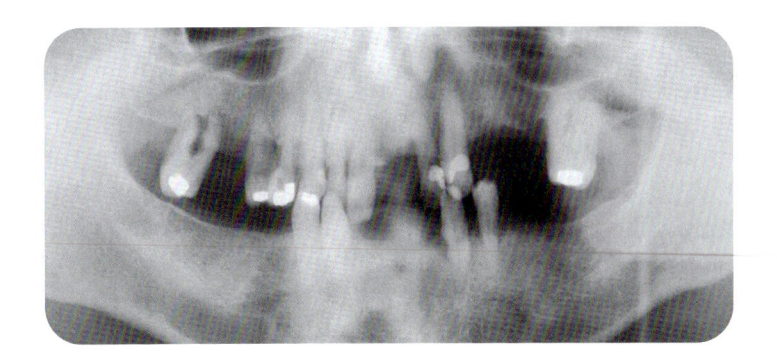

This 50-year-old man complained of a three-month history of pain related to 17. His sleep was not disturbed by the toothache, but the tooth was tender when he bit together. He did not wear upper or lower dentures. His medical history is marked by insulin dependent-diabetes mellitus and angina; he is currently taking isosorbide mononitrate, aspirin, lipoton, atenolol, humalog and humulin.

Question 1:
Discuss his dental state as demonstrated by the OPT.

Question 2:
What treatment does this patient require?

Question 3:
Why is this patient taking aspirin, and how does aspirin achieve its effects?

Explanation 1:
The OPT shows a partially dentate mouth. General bone architecture appears normal. There is generalised alveolar bone loss. Gross calculus deposits can be seen on all teeth. There is evidence of past restoration of root caries, and there are cavities in 22 and 13. The 17 has nearly 90% bone loss and an associated periapical radiolucency. It is significantly over-erupted. In addition, there appears to be a radiolucency around the apex of 12. The most likely diagnosis for this patient's pain is an acute periodontal abscess of the 17, secondary to advanced chronic adult periodontitis.

Explanation 2:
This patient does not appear to have been a regular dental attender and is unlikely to be willing to undergo any extensive treatment. The main priority with his medical history is to remove any source of pain and infection from his mouth and attempt to improve his masticatory function, as diet is an important factor in the control of diabetes.
- Extraction of 17, 12, 22 and 27 under local anaesthetic.
- Treatment of caries 13.
- Supragingival scaling and oral hygiene instruction.
- Diet advice and prescription of daily fluoride mouthwashes.
- Construction of partial upper and lower acrylic dentures onto which additional teeth can be added as required.
- Reinforcement of oral hygiene and diet advice and regular review every six months.

Explanation 3:
This patient has a history of angina, which is the discomfort due to transient myocardial ischaemia. The commonest cause for this is coronary atheroma. One sequelae of atheromatous narrowing of vessels is the formation of thrombi, which form by the aggregation of platelets and fibrin. As a preventative approach to thrombus formation patients are often prescribed anti-platelet drugs such as aspirin to prevent platelet aggregation. Aspirin is a non-steroidal anti-inflammatory drug. It acts by irreversibly inhibiting cyclo-oxygenase, thereby preventing the production of endoperoxides from arachidonic acid. The net effect is the inhibition of prostaglandin, prostacyclin and platelet thromboxane A2 (TXA-2) production. TXA-2 is a powerful stimulator of platelet aggrega-

tion and normally is antagonised by prostacyclin, which is produced by both vascular endothelial cells and platelets. Platelets are unable to produce new cyclo-oxygenase once it has been inhibited by aspirin, but vascular endothelial cells can, and therefore there is a net shift from platelet aggregation by TXA-2 to platelet disaggregation by prostacyclin.

Case 13 Dental pain

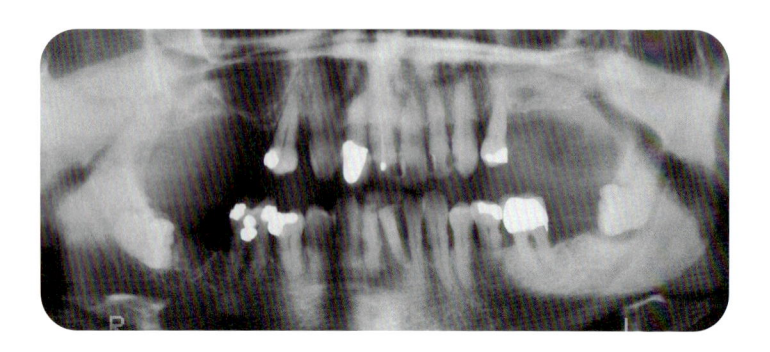

This 65-year-old man was complaining of increasing pain in the upper left quadrant, which had been getting worse over the past two weeks. He has ischaemic heart disease and hypertension and suffered a myocardial infarct six years ago. He is taking aspirin, atenolol, bendrofluazide, lisinopril, amlodipine and glyceryl trinitrate spray.

Question 1:
An OPT was taken. What do you think is the cause of his symptoms?

Question 2:
If you decide to extract teeth, in view of his medical history are there any precautions you might take?

Question 3:
What is your management for a bleeding socket in this patient?

Question 4:
What other oral disease does this patient have?

Part I – Case 13

Explanation 1:
There is an angular bony defect associated with the 25, which has lost a considerable amount of its bony support. The symptoms, together with the radiological appearance, suggest that the most likely diagnoses include either a periapical or periodontal abscess as a result of the existing perio-endo lesion.

Explanation 2:
The medical history of hypertension and anti-platelet medication predisposes this patient to an increased risk of postoperative bleeding. It is therefore advisable to carry out the extraction in the morning when blood pressure is normally lower and to take the patient's blood pressure before the extraction. If the diastolic blood pressure is 100 or above, it would be advisable not to proceed unless symptoms are very severe. Because the patient is taking aspirin, there are two possible options that can be taken:
- Have sutures and haemostatic agents at hand in case haemostasis is not easily achievable.
- With the advice of the patient's GMP, stop the aspirin four days before the extraction if you are very worried about the risk of bleeding or if the patient has had a previous episode of post-extraction bleeding.

Explanation 3:
- Ensure that constant pressure has been applied to the socket for at least 10 minutes with a roll of gauze.
- Inspect the area for signs of mucosal tears. In the absence of any tears continue pressure for a further 10 minutes. If tears are found they should be sutured.
- If bleeding still continues, place a tight mattress suture over the socket.
- If the suture is not successful, place a resorbable haemostatic agent into the socket and re-suture the wound – for instance, with oxidised cellulose.

- Give the patient clear postoperative instructions to minimise the risk of bleeding and provide emergency contact details to use in the event of any further bleeding.

Explanation 4:
There is generalised alveolar bone loss and extensive calculus deposits visible. These are suggestive of periodontal disease.

Case 14 Complications of unerupted teeth

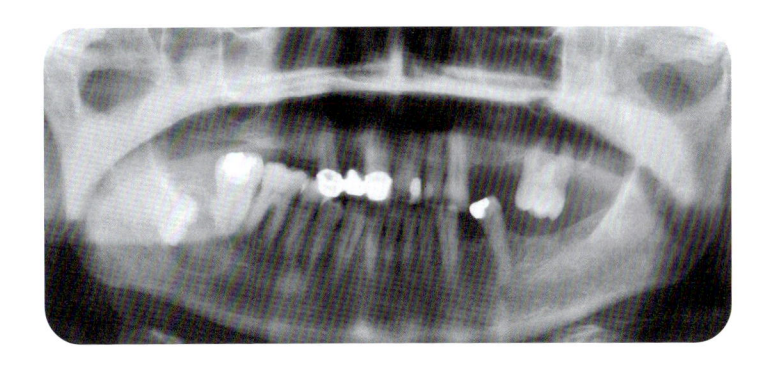

This 68-year-old woman presented with pain and aching in the lower right quadrant. She is a regular dental attender. Her medical history is marked by asthma, bronchitis and peptic ulceration. She is taking lansoprazole, salbutamol and beclomethasone dipropionate.

Question 1:
What abnormality can be seen in the OPT that was taken at this visit?

Question 2:
What are the most likely diagnoses?

Question 3:
What treatment should be provided?

Question 4:
What are the recognised indications for this treatment option?

Question 5:
What are the possible complications associated with this treatment?[19–27]

Explanation 1:
The OPT shows a partially dentate mouth. There is an unerupted, mesioangularly impacted lower right 8, the crown of which appears to be associated with a unilocular, well-defined radiolucency.

Explanation 2:
- Dentigerous cyst.
- Odontogenic keratocyst.
- Ameloblastoma.

Explanation 3:
Having obtained the fully informed consent of the patient, surgically extract the lower right 8 and the associated lesion. The specimen should be sent in formol-saline for pathological analysis.

Explanation 4:
According to the NICE guidelines 2000,[19] indications for removal of unerupted third molar teeth are:
- Any symptomatic wisdom tooth, especially where there have been one or more episodes of infection such as pericoronitis, cellulites or untreatable pulpal/periapical pathology.
- Caries where the tooth is unlikely to be usefully restored or caries in the adjacent molar, which cannot be satisfactorily treated without removal of the third molar.
- Periodontal disease due to the position of the third molar and its association with the second molar tooth.
- Pathology associated with the tooth.
- Tooth in the line of a fracture and open to the oral cavity.
- External resorption of the third molar or of the second molar where this would appear to be caused by the third molar.
- Prior to orthognathic surgery.

Part I – Case 14

Explanation 5:

Intraoperative	Postoperative
Failed LA.	Pain.
Haemorrhage.	Swelling.
Fractured root apex.	Bruising.
Damage to adjacent tooth/ soft tissue.	Trismus.
Damage to adjacent restorations.	Damage to inferior dental/lingual nerve.
Fracture of the mandible.	Infection of soft tissue/bone.

Case 15 Facial trauma

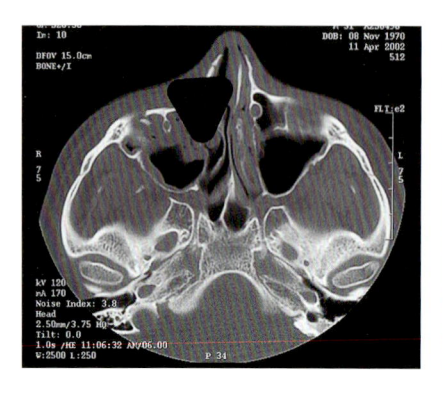

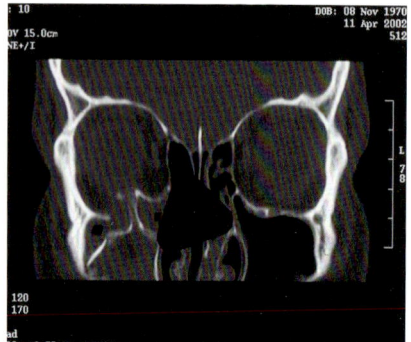

This 30-year-old man sustained a blow to his face one year ago. He did not seek treatment at the time of injury but is now complaining of diplopia and blurred vision. He is fit and well with no allergies and is not taking any prescribed medication.

Question 1:
What investigation has been performed?

Question 2:
How is this image produced?

Question 3:
What clinical feature of note can be seen in this image?

Question 4:
What are the possible the reasons for this patient's double vision?

Question 5:
What parts of the orbit are most commonly involved in such an injury?

Question 6:
What are the principles in the treatment of this patient's injury?

Part I – Case 15

Explanation 1:
A computerised tomographic (CT) scan.

Explanation 2:
A CT image is produced as a series of sectional X-ray images. The patient is placed into a tube lined with sensitive gas or crystal detectors. An X-ray tubehead is situated on the inner aspect of the detector tube. The detector records the intensity of the X-ray beam that emerges from the patient. This information is then converted into digital data, which is transmitted to a computer for conversion into an image based on a grey scale, which represents different tissue densities.

Explanation 3:
There is a comminuted fracture through the floor of the right orbit with upward displacement of the anterior fragment of the orbital floor. The right maxillary antrum is markedly opacified, suggestive of bony fragments from the antral wall.

Explanation 4:
Diplopia following traumatic injury may be the sequela of:
- An alteration in globe position – for instance, proptosis/enophthalmos.
- Limitation of the globe movement through entrapment of orbital rim soft tissues and/or the inferior rectus muscle.
- Nerve injury, either intracranially or intraorbitally, as a result of compression from haematoma or bone fragments.

Explanation 5:
This is a blow-out fracture where the sudden rise in orbital pressure causes fracture of the weakest walls of the orbital floor and medial wall. These are made up of the orbital lamina of the ethmoid bone, the lacrimal bone and the orbital surfaces of the maxilla and zygoma.

Explanation 6:
- Obtain a preoperative baseline Hess chart to assess preoperative visual field disturbance. Herztel exophthalmometry will quantify the degree of any enophthalmos.

45

- Surgically explore the fractured orbital floor and, following correct replacement of orbital contents, reduce the fracture and fixate the segments with fracture plates. Cover any residual defects in the floor of the orbit with materials such as autogenous bone, titanium mesh, specialist titianium fracture plates or a silastic sheet to prevent the contents of the orbit from being displaced into the antrum again.
- Perform eye observations for 24 hours following surgery, keeping close observation for retrobulbar bleeding.
- Review one week after discharge and obtain a postoperative Hess chart to compare pre- and post-operative visual fields.

Case 16 Sore gums

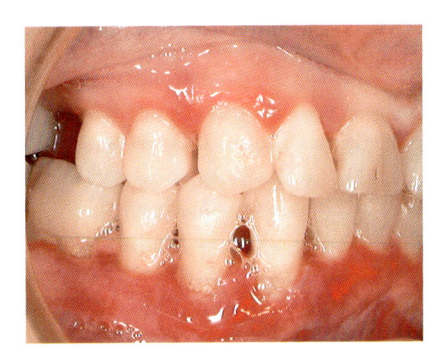

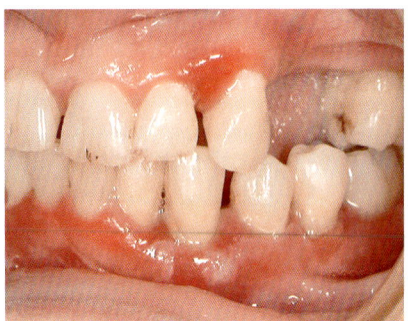

This 48-year-old patient gave a one-year history of sore, bleeding, 'peeling' gums. She has a history of eczema but is taking no prescribed medication.

Question 1:
Describe what you can see in these photographs.

Question 2:
The most likely explanation for the appearance of the gingivae is desquamative gingivitis; what conditions are associated with desquamative gingivitis?

Question 3:
How can a definitive diagnosis be made?

Question 4:
What treatment can be given to this patient?

Explanation 1:
There is marked generalised erythema of the gingivae with evidence of sloughing of the mucosa. There are no areas of ulceration or bullae on either buccal or palatal mucosae. There is evidence of early gingival recession, especially in the posterior quadrants.

Explanation 2:
- Lichen planus.
- Drug-induced lichenoid reactions.
- Menopause, related to hormonal changes.
- Cicatricial pemphigoid.
- Pemphigoid.
- Pemphigus.
- Psoriasis.
- Contact sensitivity – for instance, to toothpaste.
- Systemic or discoid lupus erythematosus (SLE or DLE).

Explanation 3:
- A thorough history needs to be taken.
- A close examination is necessary of all the clinical features present, both orally and elsewhere – for instance, on the skin.
- Gingival biopsy and histopathology of the sample.
- Direct and indirect immunofluorescence.
- Patch-testing if contact sensitivity is suspected.
- Chest X-ray if sarcoidosis is suspected.

Explanation 4:
- Try to ascertain whether there is a local agent/cause for the gingivitis by taking a thorough drug history and examination. If this does not produce an obvious cause, consider carrying out a mucosal biopsy and a haematological autoantibody screen to exclude any of the possible autoimmune causes for this disorder.
- Careful debridement and oral hygiene with adjunctive chlorhexidine gluconate mouthwash.

- Local occlusive steroid cream – for instance, fluocinolone acetonide administered via an acrylic splint for 15 minutes twice daily plus or minus adjunctive oral antibiotics – for instance, doxycycline.
- If the condition does not improve, consider prednisolone or betamethasone mouthwashes and later systemic corticosteroids.

Case 17 Mandibular radiolucency

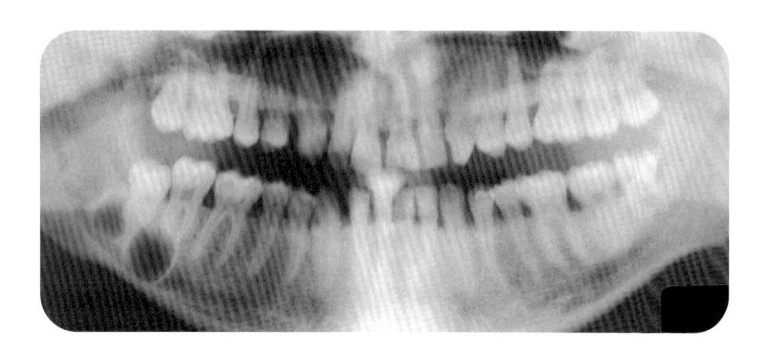

This 27-year-old man presented for a routine dental check-up. He complained of a slight ache on the right side of his jaw. He was apyrexial, with no obvious extraoral swelling. Intraorally 47 and 48 were tender to percussion, but there was no sign of decay and no notable swelling bucco-lingually. The patient was fit and well and not taking any prescribed medication.

Question 1:
What abnormal feature is present on this radiograph?

Question 2:
The lesion is diagnosed as an odontogenic keratocyst. It is surgically enucleated and the patient complains of numbness of his lip and chin following surgery. What types of injury could have occurred to the inferior dental nerve during surgery?

Question 3:
What is the clinical management of the sensory loss to this patient?

Question 4:
How often should the patient be reviewed and for how long?

Explanation 1:
The OPT shows an extensive multilocular radiolucency on the right side of the mandible located close to 47 and 48. It extends mesiodistally from the mesial root of the 47 to the sigmoid notch of the mandibular ramus and appears to be intimately related to the inferior dental canal. It is well corticated with no sign of calcific contents. There does not appear to be any resorption of the root of either 47 or 48.

Explanation 2:
- *Neuropraxia* – where there is mild insult to the nerve, resulting in conduction disruption. There is no axonal degeneration and sensory recovery is complete in a matter of hours to several days. Clinically usually manifests as paraesthesia.
- *Axonotmesis* – where there is a more severe injury to the nerve, axonal fibre degeneration occurs. This is common in nerve stretching. The nerve is still however, grossly intact and recovery is usually good, if incomplete, after a period of a few months. It manifests as severe paraesthesia or anaesthesia.
- *Neurotmesis* – here the nerve is completely severed or disrupted, and recovery is not usually expected. However, because the inferior alveolar nerve is located in a canal the fibres do occasionally regenerate to give a little recovery of sensation, which is incomplete.

Explanation 3:
In all cases of nerve damage it must be borne in mind that any recovery is time-dependent. Therefore the initial management should be to map out the exact location and nature of neurosensory deficit and to follow up the patient at regular intervals for three months to observe any change over time. If there has been no improvement at all after this period, an attempt can be made to repair the damaged nerve microneurosurgically. Before embarking on this type of surgery, the patient should be warned that improvement is not guaranteed by surgery, and sensory loss may well persist. They must also be warned that in some cases dysaesthesia may develop.

Explanation 4:

Because of the nerve injury this patient should be reviewed every month for three months until a decision is made to repair the nerve or to accept the situation and see if some recovery takes place; this may take up to 18 months.[28] Because the lesion removed was an odontogenic keratocyst, the patient should be reviewed yearly for the next eight to ten years due to the high recurrence rate.

Case 18 Dental trauma

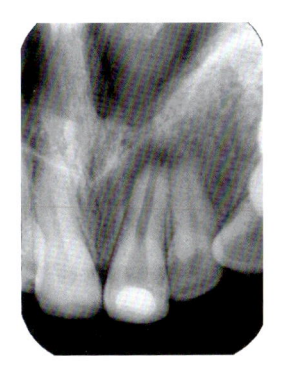

A 17-year-old girl complained of an unsightly 11 related to a traumatic injury nine years earlier. A clinical examination was carried out and intraoral periapical and standard occlusal radiographs were taken. There was a suppurating sinus buccal to 11, which is grade II mobile. The patient is fit and well and not taking any prescribed medication.

Question 1:
What do you think is the cause of her symptoms?

Question 2:
How would you manage this case clinically?

Question 3:
The tooth was treated endodontically initially, but the crown fractured and the suppurating sinus persisted despite a satisfactory root filling. The 11 was subsequently extracted and it has now been decided to place an implant. There is, however, a significant bony defect as a result of the previous chronic infection. What options are there for implant placement here?

Question 4:
How long should the first stage implant be left before it can be loaded?

Question 5:
What is osseointegration?

Question 6:
How can you test for osseointegration?

Explanation 1:
The periapical radiograph shows an area of internal resorption in the crown of the 11, the apex of 11 is incomplete and open and there is a periapical radiolucency suggestive of a periapical abscess which is the most likely cause for the mobility and draining sinus.

Explanation 2:
There are several treatment options possible for this case.
- Pulp extirpation and dressing of the pulp canal with non-setting calcium hydroxide dressings every three months until there is no further sign of progression of resorption. The canal can then be obturated with gutta percha.
- Extraction of the tooth and replacement of the tooth with either a resin-bonded bridge or an osseointegrated implant and crown.

Explanation 3:
Bony defects can be filled using a bone graft. The location of graft harvest depends largely on the amount of bone required. For a single implant site, an easily accessible source of bone is the retromolar area. The implant can then be placed directly into the grafted bone. Other potential donor autograft sites include iliac crest, rib, tibia and calvaria. Other options include using allograft, xenograft, alloplastic materials or a combination.

Explanation 4:
Ideally an implant should be allowed to osseointegrate before functional loading. Sufficient time for osseointegration to occur is influenced by many factors, such as bone quality.

Explanation 5:
Osseointegration is the direct apposition of bone against the implant surface without the presence of any fibrous tissue between bone and implant.

Explanation 6:
- Percussion of the implant.
- Testing for immobility of the implant.
- Torque testing.
- USS frequency.

Case 19 Dental pain

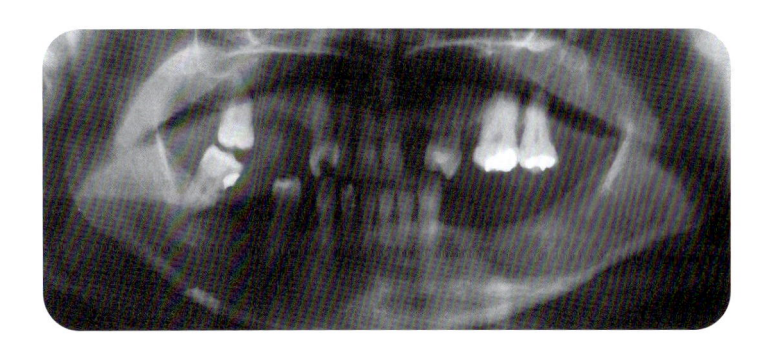

This 45-year-old woman presented with intermittent pain of four weeks' duration on the right side of her mandible. The pain was exacerbated by eating, drinking and lasted for over 30 minutes. An OPT was taken.

Question 1:
What do you think may be the cause of her symptoms?

Question 2:
What other abnormal features are there of note on the OPT?

Question 3:
This patient suffers from thyrotoxicosis. What are the causes for this and what are the associated clinical features?[29,30]

Question 4:
If you decide to carry out extractions as the first part of your treatment plan, would this patient's thyroid disease have any implications?

Question 5:
What other treatment does this patient require?

55

Explanation 1:
There is a large carious lesion in the 48 and a radiolucent area around its apex, possibly the result of a combination of advanced periodontal disease and periapical infection. The symptoms this patient is suffering are likely to be related to an irreversible pulpitis of the 48, secondary to caries.

Explanation 2:
There is generalised recession of alveolar bone with angular defects around the roots of 17, 26 and 48. This patient appears to be suffering from advanced chronic adult periodontitis.

There is a large cavity in the 15, which may be due to either caries or a lost restoration. The 42 has been crowned; there is an apical radiolucency associated with this tooth. This is likely to be a chronic periapical granuloma or abscess.

Explanation 3:
Causes: Graves' disease, toxic multinodular goitre, adenoma, acute thyroiditis, metastatic thyroid carcinoma, TSH-secreting tumour.

Clinical features: weight loss, increased appetite, irritability, muscle weakness, tremor, heat intolerance, palpitations, eye signs, goitre, hyperkinesis, psychosis, tachycardia, proximal myopathy, vasodilated peripheries, pretibial myxoedema.

Explanation 4:
- This patient is likely to be anxious/irritable during the procedure, so treatment should involve as little pain as possible.
- There is a theoretical risk that the use of adrenaline-containing anaesthetic carries the risk of exacerbating any pre-existing tachycardia. However, there is no clinical evidence to either contraindicate the used of adrenaline or proof that any other agent is safer.

Explanation 5:
- Full periodontal assessment with supragingival scaling initially. Give oral hygiene instruction to assess the patient's motivation to achieve better oral health. If she responds well to basic periodontal treat-

ment consider deep scaling and root planing in an attempt to control the periodontal disease.
- Vitality test 15 and 42. Restore with or without RCT, depending on the clinical findings.
- Construct partial dentures to replace missing teeth. Consider implants at this stage
- Review the patient at three-monthly intervals to reinforce oral hygiene instruction.

Case 20 Xerostomia

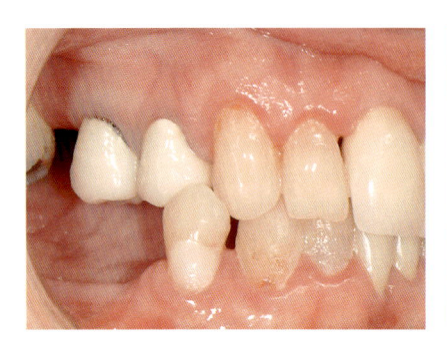

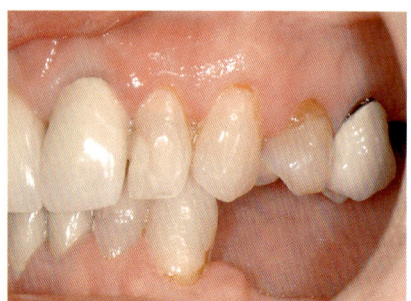

This 60-year-old woman complained of a severely dry mouth and difficulty in tolerating her lower partial denture. She had had extensive dental treatment and was a regular attender at the dental surgery. Her medical history comprises systemic lupus erythematosus (SLE) and Sjögren's syndrome.

Question 1:
What is systemic lupus erythematosus and how may it present in the oral cavity?

Question 2:
What are the implications of SLE in dental treatment?

Question 3:
Using the history and photographs what treatment do you think this patient requires?

Question 4:
If she is still not able to tolerate a partial denture despite providing a new well-fitting one, what would you do?

Explanation 1:
Systemic lupus erythematosus (SLE) is a multisystem connective tissue disease characterised by the presence of numerous autoantibodies, circulating immune complexes and widespread immunologically determined tissue damage. Oral manifestations are:
- Mucosal lesions on buccal mucosa and lips. Comprised of a central depressed red atrophic area surrounded by an elevated keratotic zone that dissolves into white striae. Occasionally there is ulceration. Easily confused with lichen planus lesions.
- Over 75% of SLE patients have oral complaints of burning mouth, xerostomia or soreness.

Explanation 2:
- Thrombocytopenia may be severe and a platelet count should be performed before surgery.
- SLE patients are predisposed to the development of Libman-Sacks vegetations under the mitral valve, which can lead to bacterial endocarditis. Therefore any SLE patient with a heart murmur should have antibiotic prophylaxis for any procedure likely to cause a significant bacteraemia.
- SLE can be exacerbated by NSAIDs, penicillin and sulphonamides. These should be avoided where possible.
- SLE can be exacerbated by surgery. Elective surgery should therefore be avoided where possible.
- SLE patients are often taking high-dose long-term corticosteroids and therefore are susceptible to shock and infection.

Explanation 3:
- Restoration of carious dentition and failed restorations – 15, 45, 32, 33, 42, 43 and 44.
- Prescribe fluoride mouthwashes. Consider prescribing saliva substitute.
- Assess for a construction of a new partial lower denture.
- Regular recall to monitor control of caries rate and assess tolerance of dentures.

Explanation 4:

Options to restore spaces are to construct bridgework or place implants. The main problem with putting bridgework into this patient's mouth is the high caries rate. If this can be stabilised then bridgework may well be possible. Implant surgery would be stressful and should be undertaken only by an experienced surgeon as part of an experienced care team.

Case 21 Retained roots

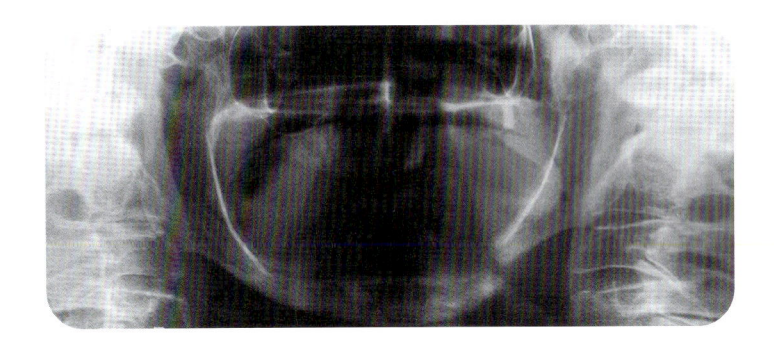

A 65-year-old woman presented with a sublingual space abscess related to a retained infected 25 root. Her medical history was marked by thyrotoxicosis, angina, emphysema and osteoarthritis. She is taking ipratropium bromide, beclomethasone dipropionate, and prednisolone.

Question 1:
What are the boundaries and contents of the sublingual space?

Question 2:
What is the management of this sublingual space abscess?

Question 3:
Following treatment of the infection, the patient complained of persistent pain and an inability to wear her lower full denture. The OPT was taken at this appointment. What was the cause of her symptoms?

Question 4:
What are the treatment options?

Explanation 1:
The sublingual space lies above the mylohyoid muscle. The roof is made up of the floor of the mouth mucosa and the floor is bounded by the mylohyoid, genioglossus, gleniohyoid, styloglossus, tongue and lingual frenum. This space contains the sublingual glands, which wrap around the lingual frenum. There are also the vessels and nerves supplying these glands, namely the sublingual, submental arteries and branches of the lingual and chorda tympani nerves.

Explanation 2:
Any infection of the floor of the mouth is potentially a risk to the patient's airway. Treatment involves prompt incision and drainage of the abscess and removal of the source, which, in this case, involves extraction of the retained, infected 25 root. This can be achieved via an intraoral approach taking care not to damage one of the sublingual glands, the submandibular duct or the lingual nerve.

Explanation 3:
There is a displaced fracture of the mandibular body in the region where the root was extracted. This is a pathological fracture, which has occurred because the mandible is atrophic and edentulous and the surgery has weakened the substance of the remaining bone.

Explanation 4:
The fact that this patient has already had a general anaesthetic very recently combined with her complex medical history puts her at high risk of developing serious post-general anaesthetic respiratory complications. The first approach therefore in the management of this fracture could be to see if it will heal conservatively without surgical intervention and to reline the lower full denture to increase its stability. She should be advised to eat a very soft diet. If in one month's time there has been no satisfactory union of the fracture, the only option is to treat the fracture surgically. Although there are a number of options,[31-33] the most favoured ones in such a clinical situation are:
- Open reduction and internal rigid fixation.
- Rib-grafting and plating.

Case 22 Facial sinus

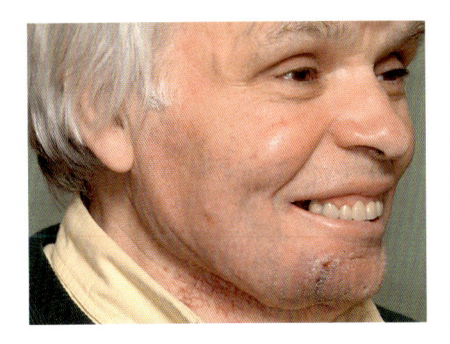

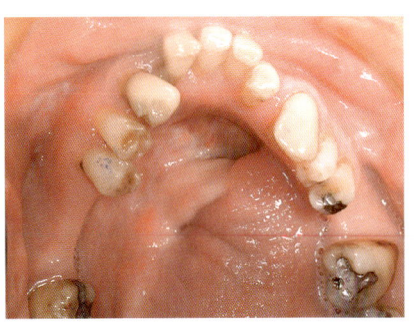

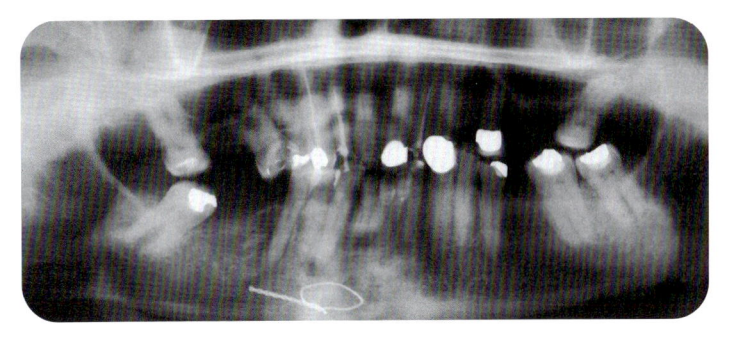

This 60-year-old man complained of a three-month history of a suppurating sinus on his chin. Seven years ago he underwent resection of a squamous cell carcinoma of the floor of mouth with reconstruction, using a radial forearm microvascular free flap. He received postoperative radiotherapy. He is not taking any medication and has no known allergies.

Question 1:
What do you think may be the aetiology of the sinus?

Question 2:
How would you treat this case?

Question 3:
Which are the most appropriate antibiotics to prescribe to this patient post-operatively and what is the mechanism of their action?

Explanation 1:
The photograph shows the sinus to be located parallel to the lower right canine region and adjacent to a fracture wire in the mandible. Although not very clear on the OPT, there appear to be radiolucencies around the apices of the 42 and 43 which may relate to areas of infection. The crowns of the lower incisors appear to be significantly reduced in size, possibly due to parafunction. The most likely source of infection is therefore either the wire or the 42 or 43, which may have become non-vital either as a result of the radiotherapy or from occlusal trauma.

Explanation 2:
Because of this patient' history of radiotherapy to this region, infection of any source is at high risk of poor healing and could potentially lead to osteomyelitis. The management of this patient should therefore be centred around removing/treating any potential source of infection. To minimise potential trauma, root canal therapy should be performed in favour of extraction of the 42 and 43. In addition, the border wire should be removed surgically. This may be done with preoperative hyperbaric oxygen and postoperative broad-spectrum antibiotics to minimise the chances of the development of osteoradionecrosis.

Explanation 3:
Ideally the antibiotic of choice should be one that acts specifically on bacteria cultured from a wound swab preoperatively. If this has not been done, the best choice of antibiotic is either a broad-spectrum antibiotic such as co-amoxiclav or a combination of amoxycillin and metronidazole, which would act against both gram-positive aerobic and anaerobic gram-negative bacteria. Amoxycillin is a broad-spectrum penicillin. It is bactericidal and acts by preventing cross-linkage between peptidoglycan polymer chains in bacterial cell walls. It is effective against non-β lactamase-producing gram-positive bacteria as well as some gram-negative bacteria.

Metronidazole belongs to the 5-nitroimidazole group of antibacterial drugs. They act by diffusing into organisms and reducing nitro groups. The products of this reduction process inhibit DNA synthesis and/or damage the DNA thus impairing its function. It is active against anaerobic bacteria and some protozoa.

Case 23 Chance findings on an OPT

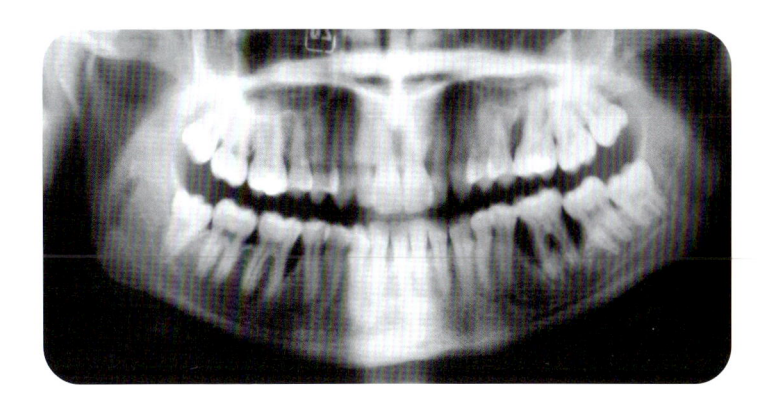

This 15-year-old girl was referred by her orthodontist for an opinion about an unusual finding in her pre-orthodontic treatment OPT and periapical radiographs. She is fit and well and not taking any medication.

Question 1:
What is unusual about the radiograph?

Question 2:
What is the cause of this condition?

Question 3:
How is this condition treated?

Question 4:
This girl wishes to undergo orthodontic treatment. Do you think that this is an appropriate case for orthodontics?

Question 5:
What systemic conditions have been implicated in the aetiology of this condition?

Explanation 1:
The periapical radiographs show prominent angular bone loss that appears to be symmetrically affecting all of the first molar teeth. These findings are suggestive of a diagnosis of localised aggressive periodontitis (LAP).[34,35]

Explanation 2:
The aetiology of LAP is believed to be a combination of genetic predisposition and specific bacterial infection. The bony defect is probably genetically determined. There are a number of organisms that have been cultured from the pockets in LAP, but *Actinobacillus actinomycetemcomitans* is the main pathogen, cultured from over 90% of pockets. Other implicated organisms include *Capnocytophaga sp.*, *Eikenella corrodens* and *Bacteroides sp*.

Explanation 3:
- In severe cases teeth may need to be extracted.
- In early disease attempts can be made to control its progression through meticulous oral hygiene and regular scaling.
- Pockets should be root-planed to remove all pathogenic organisms and toxins. Flap surgery may be required to ensure good access.
- Antimicrobial treatment can be highly effective in the early stages of this disease. The best agent to prescribe is a tetracycline, given for a two- to three-week course in conjunction with the above intervention.

Explanation 4:
Localised periodontitis is not *per se* a definitive contraindication to orthodontic treatment. The most important factor is that the patient is compliant and able to carry out meticulous oral hygiene and is willing to attend two-monthly regular hygiene appointments throughout any orthodontic treatment. It would be wise to carry out OHI, scaling, root-planing and antimicrobial treatment before orthodontic treatment begins and to monitor the response to treatment.

Explanation 5:
- Immunodeficiencies:
  - Down syndrome.
  - Leukopenia.
  - Severe uncontrolled diabetes mellitus.
  - HIV infection.

- Genetic syndromes:
  - Hypophosphatasia.
  - Papillon-Lefèvre syndrome.
  - Type VIII Ehlers Danlos syndrome.
  - Eosinophilic granuloma.

Case 24 Sore mouth

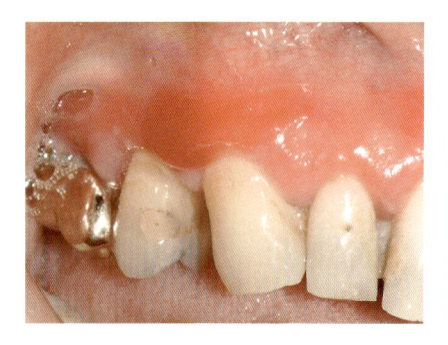

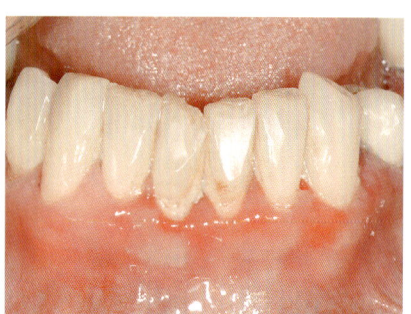

This 50-year-old man complained of a sore mouth and blood blisters on his gums. These symptoms had been present for two years but were getting worse. His medication includes ramipril, atenolol, amlodipine, frusemide, atorvastatin, aspirin, lansoprazole and glycerol trinitrate spray (GTN).

Question 1:
What abnormal features can you see in the photographs?

Question 2:
What condition does this clinical picture resemble?

Question 3:
What disorders can present in the mouth with similar lesions?

Question 4:
How are the most common bullous lesions differentiated histologically?

Question 5:
What is the difference between direct and indirect immunofluorescence?

Part I – Case 24

Explanation 1:
There is evidence of blistering around the gingival margins as well as some healing erosions. There are no striations, scars or white patches visible and there is no evidence of sloughing of mucosa. There is a visible collection of plaque around the gingival margins.

Explanation 2:
The presence of intact bullae and multiple erosions present for a period of years suggests the presence of a vesiculobullous disorder, such as mucous membrane pemphigoid.

Explanation 3:
- Pemphigus vulgaris and vegetans.
- Viral infections (such as herpes zoster).
- Cicatricial pemphigoid.
- Dermatitis herpetiformis.
- Bullous lichen planus.
- Epidermolysis bullosa.
- Erythema multiforme.

Explanation 4:
Pemphigus is characterised by the presence of *intraepithelial bullae* and cleft-like spaces produced by acantholysis. These changes occur between stratum spinosum cells just above the basal layer. There is little inflammatory cell infiltration. Direct immunofluorescence shows the presence of IgG autoantibody bound to the surface of prickle cells. In contrast, pemphigoid is characterised by the presence of *subepithelial bullae*. There is separation of the full thickness of the epithelium from the lamina propria. There is development of mainly lymphocytic infiltration in the lamina propria as the vesicle enlarges. Direct immunofluorescence show the presence of IgG autoantibody bound along the basement membrane

Explanation 5:
Immunofluorescence is a technique that uses the highly specific binding between antibodies and antigens to diagnose disease. In direct immunofluorescence, fluorescent-labelled anti-IgG antibody is added to a section of fresh frozen tissue on a microscope slide. This is then left

to incubate, thus allowing any IgG in the specimen to bind to the anti-IgG antibodies. The excess is then washed off and the specimen is viewed under an ultraviolet-light microscope. In contrast with indirect immunofluorescence, a drop of the patient's serum is added to a section of his own tissue on a slide. Fluorescent-labelled anti-IgG antibody is then added and the sample incubated. The specimen is then viewed under an ultraviolet light microscope. In essence, direct immunofluorescence is a method of detecting autoantibodies in tissue, whereas indirect immunofluorescence detects circulating autoantibodies in serum.

Case 25 White patch

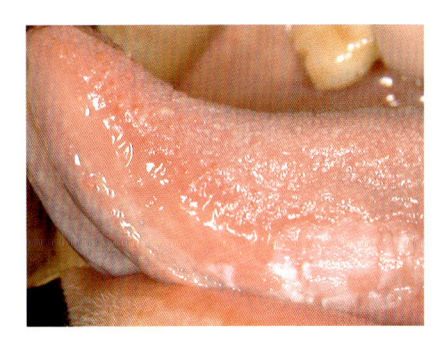

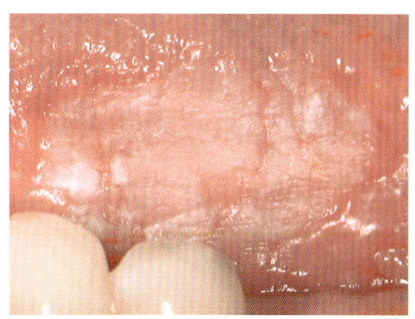

This 76-year-old woman was concerned about a white patch on her tongue. She had been aware of its presence for the past four years but was worried because it had started to grow and had changed in appearance. She had not experienced pain from the area. She suffers from arthritis for which she is taking regular ibuprofen. She is a non-smoker and drinks less than 10 units of alcohol per week.

Question 1:
Describe the clinical features of the lesion.

Question 2:
Give your differential diagnosis for the lesion shown in this photograph.

Question 3:
What are the risk factors which would increase the chances of leukoplakia undergoing malignant change?[36]

Question 4:
What are the management principles for this lesion?

Explanation 1:
The photograph shows a white area on the lateral border of the tongue measuring approximately 2cm in length. The area appears to be raised and non-ulcerated. There are no interspersed areas of erythema and it has a non-erythematous margin.

Explanation 2:

(Traumatic)	mechanical (frictional keratosis)
	thermal
(Infective)	candidosis – chronic hyperplastic
(Idiopathic)	leukoplakia
(Dermatological)	lichen planus
	lupus erythematosus
(Neoplastic)	dysplasia
	carcinoma *in situ*
	squamous cell carcinoma

Explanation 3:
- Excessive alcohol intake.
- Betel nut chewing habits.
- Site of lesion (highest risk floor of mouth, ventral tongue, lingual aspect of lower alveolar mucosa).
- Degree of dysplasia.
- Chronic anaemia.
- Interspersed erythroplakia.
- Candidal infection.
- Smoking.
- Genetic predisposition.

Explanation 4:
- Biopsy to assess degree of dysplasia.
- Test for candidal infection, anaemia and treat accordingly.
- Assess risk of malignant change based on clinical and histological assessment.
- Consider surgical excision of lesion.
- Review the patient three- to six-monthly to observe for malignant change.

Case 26 TMJ problems

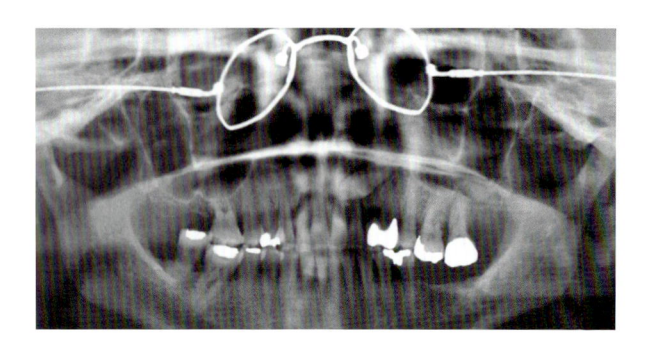

An 80-year-old man presented with pain, limitation and clicking of his right temporomandibular joint on opening and eating. These symptoms started suddenly one week ago. On examination, he had right TMJ clicking on opening, normal lateral movements but a deviation to the right side on opening. There was marked limitation of opening, which had a maximal limit of 10mm. There was no tenderness of the muscles of mastication but the right TMJ was tender to palpation. He admitted to grinding his teeth when sleeping. He has epilepsy which is controlled, a history of a stroke and atrial fibrillation.

Question 1:
What is the most likely cause for his symptoms?

Question 2:
How is this condition managed?

Question 3:
How do rheumatoid arthritis and osteoarthritis differ clinically?

Question 4:
What are the radiological differences between osteoarthritis and rheumatoid arthritis?

Part I – Case 26

Explanation 1:
The history of acute pain, clicking and limitation of opening associated with evidence of parafunction and a significantly reduced dental arch are highly suggestive of acute temporomandibular joint dysfunction syndrome.

Explanation 2:
- Reassure the patient of the benign nature of this disorder.
- Give advice on jaw relaxation exercises and make the patient aware of any parafunctional habits.
- Consider construction of dentures to improve masticatory function and reduce the loading of the right side.
- Recommend a soft diet and placement of a hot water bottle onto the joint and the use of simple analgesics at times of pain.
- If the above does not improve symptoms consider construction of an occlusal splint.
- In some cases antidepressants can work.
- As a last resort, surgery may be needed to correct any internal joint derangement. This would involve initially arthroscopy followed by an open arthrotomy +/- meniscopexy if there is extensive damage to the meniscus.

Explanation 3:

Osteoarthritis	Rheumatoid arthritis
Valgus, varus or flexion deformities of joints.	Involves hips, hand, wrists, feet, knees.
Heberden's and Bouchard's nodes (DI/PI joints).	PI/MCP and wrist joints swollen. Ulnar deviation, swan neck/boutonniere deformities. Multiple non-articular symptoms affecting CVS, CNS, kidneys, lungs and eyes.
Worse in evenings, and aggravated by use.	Joint pain worst in the morning.

Pain in knees, hips or hands.	Fatigue common.
Hard and bony swellings with movement crepitus.	Soft-tissue swellings.
Limitation of movement.	Tenderness on pressure/movement.

Explanation 4:

Osteoarthritis	Rheumatoid arthritis
Subchondral sclerosis.	Juxta-articular osteoporosis.
Joint space narrowing.	Joint space narrowing.
Osteophytes.	Periarticular erosions.
Subchondral cysts.	

Case 27 Facial pain

A 65-year-old woman presented with a seven-year history of severe shooting pain on the left side of her face that radiates to behind her left eye. The pain is exacerbated whenever she touches that side of her face. In addition she is also experiencing a burning sensation all over her tongue. This is a constant soreness that shows no pattern of onset. She is hypertensive and suffers from depression. She is taking frusemide, amitryptilline, and doxazocin.

Question 1:
What disorders does this patient have?

Question 2:
What special tests would you perform on this patient?

Question 3:
What is the most common drug prescibed for the facial pain?

Question 4:
What are its potential side-effects?

Question 5:
If medical treatment fails to control the pain, what is the next treatment option?

Explanation 1:
The history of the pain this patient describes on her face carries the hallmark features of trigeminal neuralgia. Other potential causes of this type of longstanding pain could be the presence of an intracranial tumour or psychogenic/atypical facial pain. The history of a burning tongue, distributed throughout the tongue, is not likely to be related to the facial pain and is suggestive of burning mouth syndrome. It must be borne in mind, however, that these symptoms can also be related to haematological deficiencies of iron, folate or B12 or the presence of candidal infection. In addition, a psychogenic cause is also possible.

Explanation 2:
- Oral rinse and imprints for candidal infection.
- Blood screen for anaemia.
- OPT to exclude potential dental/temporomandibular joint cause.
- CT/MRI scan to exclude intracranial neoplastic disease.

Explanation 3:
Carbamazepine is an anticonvulsant drug that acts by stabilising neural membranes through the reduction of sodium and potassium conductance, thereby reducing neuronal firing.

Explanation 4:
- Nausea and vomiting.
- Dizziness, drowsiness, visual disturbances, headache, confusion or psychosis.
- Constipation or diarrhoea.
- Mild transient erthematous rash, alopecia, or Stevens-Johnson syndrome.
- Leucopenia or aplastic anaemia.
- Gynaecomastia.
- Liver or renal failure.

Explanation 5:
The final resort in the management of trigeminal neuralgia is surgery.[37–39] This usually involves cryotherapy to the trigeminal nerve or cryotherapy at the base of the skull. If these fail, another option is to carry out microvascular decompression of the trigeminal ganglion.[40]

Case 28 Facial laceration

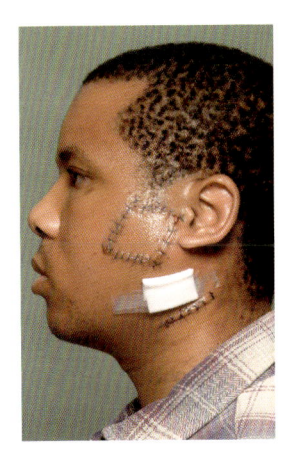

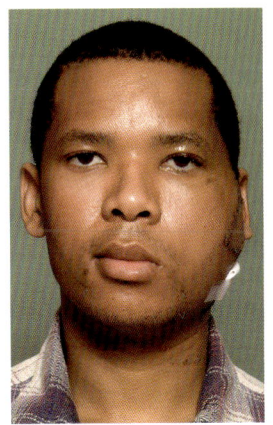

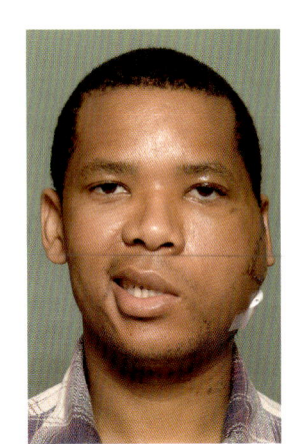

This 20-year-old patient was allegedly assaulted and suffered a laceration to the left side of his face. Medically he is fit and well.

Question 1:
Judging from the photographs, what structures were likely to have been involved in the injury?

Question 2:
The laceration extended through a gland. What gland is this, and what structures pass through this gland?

Question 3:
What nerve supplies motor stimulation to the face, and what is its course from origin to termination?

Question 4:
What short- and long-term complications may arise as a result of the injuries sustained by this patient?

Explanation 1:
The photographs show a deep rectangular laceration to the left cheek. There is weakness of the facial nerve on the left side of the face, as demonstrated by the unilateral drooping of the face. If the laceration had been full thickness it would have passed through the skin with associated adnexae, fascia, parotid gland and masseter.

Explanation 2:
The gland is the parotid salivary gland. The structures passing through from superficial to deep are:
- The facial nerve.
- The retromandibular vein.
- The external carotid artery.

Explanation 3:
The facial nerve (seventh cranial nerve):
- Arises from the facial motor nucleus in the pons.
- Leaves the pons at the cerebellopontine angle medial to CNVII as facial motor root.
- Crosses the subarachnoid space to enter the internal auditory meatus, passing laterally along it, to enter the facial canal.
- It passes onto the medial wall of the middle ear before turning 90 degrees posteriorly at the geniculate ganglion. It continues to run posteriorly until it turns 90 degrees inferiorly to run through the mastoid antrum.
- It leaves the middle ear through the stylomastoid foramen to pass between the mastoid process and the external auditory meatus.
- It enters the posterior part of the parotid gland and divides at once into superior and inferior divisions that then give rise to temporal, zygomatic, buccal, marginal mandibular and cervical branches.
- These branches emerge from the anterior periphery of the gland and lie on the surface of the masseter where they fan out over the face to supply the muscles of facial expression.

Explanation 4:
- Short-term:
  - Infection/breakdown of wound.
  - Eye infection.
  - Bleeding.
  - Dribbling.
  - Early symptoms of post-traumatic stress.

- Long-term:
  - Scarring contracture.
  - Keloid scarring.
  - Development of post-traumatic stress disorder and/or depression.

Case 29 Facial deformity

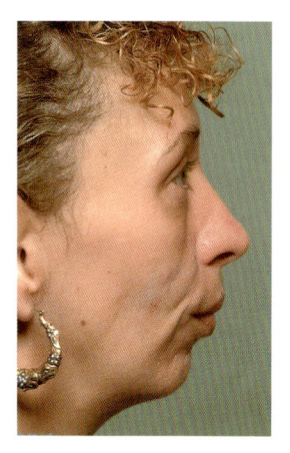

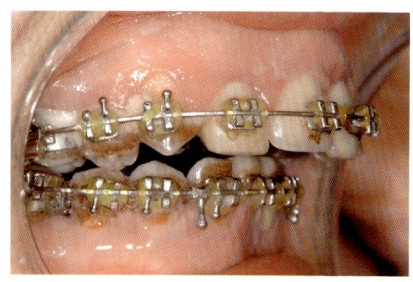

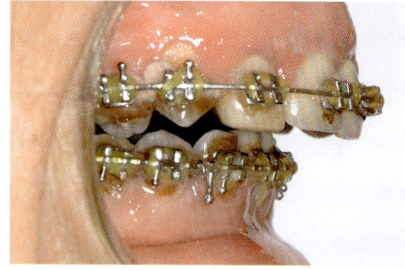

This woman was unhappy with the 'goofy' appearance of her teeth and wanted some treatment to improve this. She was a regular attender at the dental surgery and had successfully given up smoking six months earlier. She has asthma for which she takes ventolin occasionally and is allergic to penicillin.

Question 1:
Looking at the photographs, describe the dento-skeletal relationships of this patient.

Question 2:
It has been decided that a bimaxillary osteotomy is required to treat this patient. What is the purpose of the orthodontic treatment she has received?

Question 3:
What are possible specific complications of a bimaxillary osteotomy?

Explanation 1:
- Extraorally:
    - Marked class II skeletal pattern with reduced lower face height. There is no marked transverse asymmetry.
    - Lips are only competent with pursing and the upper incisors rest on the lower lip. There is a reduced nasolabial angle. Labial gingivae are visible on smiling.

- Intraorally:
    - No gross areas of plaque but some marginal gingivitis evident. Fixed orthodontic appliance in place.
    - Teeth are well aligned buccally and labially. The lower second premolars are absent, possibly extracted prior to orthodontic treatment to create space for alleviation of crowding.
    - There is a markedly increased overjet. Overbite cannot be seen in these photographs. There is a centreline shift of half a unit to the left.
    - Buccal segment are one unit class II. There is no crowding, spacing or displacement of teeth, and there are no crossbites.
    - Clinically this patient has a Class II division 1 dental relationship on a severe class II skeletal base.

Explanation 2:
This patient has undergone preorthognathic decompensation using fixed appliance orthodontics. The aim of this is to align and coordinate the arches so that the teeth will not interfere when the jaws are realigned. The teeth are moved into the ideal position, which conforms to the features of Andrew's six keys of occlusion and the dentoalveolar compensation for the skeletal discrepancy is corrected.

Explanation 3:

Intraoperative	Postoperative
Bleeding.	Relapse.
Improper maxillary/mandibular segment alignment.	Bleeding.
Unfavourable osteotomy splits.	Neurological dysfunction.
Inability to stabilise the maxilla.	Mandibular dysfunction.
Nerve injury.	Wound infection/dehiscence.
	Unfavourable facial aesthetics.

Case 30 Lump on the lip

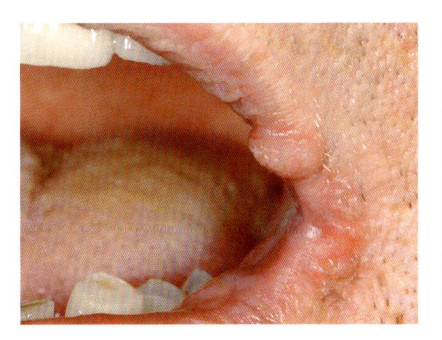

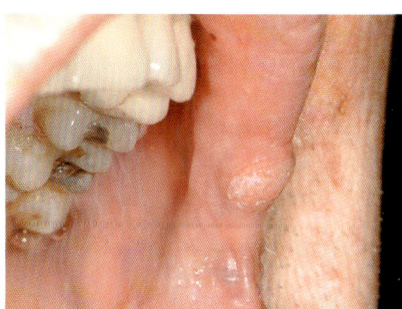

This 64-year-old man complained of a lump on his upper lip that has been present for the past four months. It was painless and had not been bleeding. He currently smokes 20 cigarettes a day. He had a renal transplant six years ago and is taking diazepam, aspirin, frusemide, cyclosporin, ranitidine, atenolol, lisinopril and prednisolone.

Question 1:
What are the photographs showing?

Question 2:
What could this be?

Question 3:
This patient has signs of gingival hyperplasia intraorally. What do you think is the cause of this?

Question 4:
What treatment would this patient require if the lesion was a squamous cell carcinoma?

Question 5:
Describe in detail how you would surgically treat this lesion.

Explanation 1:
The photographs show the left labial commissure of a man's lips. There is a raised lesion on the upper lip, approximately 2.5cm in diameter. It appears to have a central granular area and slight rolling of the margins. There is no evidence of bleeding or pigmentation.

Explanation 2:
- Fibroepithelial polyp.
- Basal cell papilloma.
- Acanthoma.
- Squamous cell carcinoma.

Explanation 3:
This patient is taking cyclosporin, an immunosuppressive drug, which has many side-effects, including gingival hyperplasia. The exact mechanism for the hyperplastic response is still not clear, but studies have suggested a role for cyclosporin in increasing fibroblast proliferation, upgrading of keratinocyte growth factor receptor expression and suppression of degradation of extracellular matrix. In addition, it has been shown that patients taking cyclosporin have a much-reduced ability to respond to the inflammatory response to subgingival plaque.[42,43]

Explanation 4:
- The diagnosis is a squamous cell carcinoma.
- Thorough examination of the neck for potential regional metastases, including CT/MRI scan and ultrasound scan of the neck.
- Surgical excision of the lip lesion with a 1cm margin of clinically normal tissue with or without a neck dissection, depending on whether or not the neck has involved nodes or not.
- Regular follow-up.
- Periodontal treatment involving deep scaling plus or minus gingival recontouring.
- Instruction in cessation of smoking habit and meticulous oral hygiene.

Explanation 5:
- Take a thorough medical history and gain informed consent from the patient.
- Excise the lesion using a wedge incision that includes a margin of around 1cm of tissue of normal appearance, preferably under local anaesthetic (in view of this patient's medical history).
- Ensure complete haemostasis.
- Place a suture at one margin to provide orientation.
- Close the defect primarily with sutures and send the specimen fixed in formol-saline for assessment of whether or not the margins are clear of tumour.
- Review after 10 days for suture removal and to arrange follow-up appointments for the future.

Case 31 Mandibular radiolucency

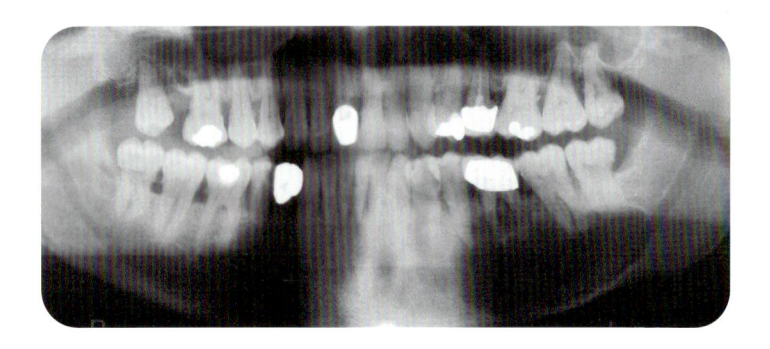

This 42-year-old man complained of pain over the left side of his mouth around his gums, which he described as a dull ache that was not worse at night or on eating. He had also noted that some of the lower teeth on that side were mobile. He is a smoker but does not drink alcohol. He has chronic bronchitis but is not taking any prescribed medication.

Question 1:
An OPT was taken. Describe what you can see in the OPT.

Question 2:
How would you ascertain a definitive diagnosis?

Question 3:
What are the histological differences between a radicular cyst and an odontogenic keratocyst?

Question 4:
What is your treatment plan for this patient?

Part I – Case 31

Explanation 1:
The OPT shows a fully dentate mouth with crowns on 11, 25, 36 and 44. The 36 has a short root filling. There is generalised alveolar bone loss and subgingival calculus suggestive of periodontal disease. The condyles and temporomandibular joints have a normal appearance on this radiograph, and the general architecture of the mandibular bone appears to be normal, except for the lower left body region where there is a large, well-defined radiolucent area. The lesion spans from 35 to 37 and occupies most of the medullary space along its length. There is no sign of calcification within the lesion. It extends into the interproximal bone between 35 and 36. There is no evidence of apical root resorption or tooth displacement associated with any of the three teeth closely related to it. The lamina durae of 35 and 36 appear to have been lost in the lesion.

Explanation 2:
Diagnosis can only be ascertained by sampling the contents of the lesion and analysing them. This can be achieved by inserting a wide-bore needle into the area and aspirating some of the contents. The sample can then be sent for pathological analysis and measurement of protein content.

Explanation 3:

	Radicular cyst	**Odontogenic keratocyst**
Origin	Epithelial rests of malassez.	Dental lamina.
Capsule	Chronically inflamed fibrous tissue. Rich vascularity. Can contain cholesterol clefts and haemosiderin deposits.	Thin friable fibrous tissue loosely attached to underlying epithelium. Occasional satellite cysts.
Lining	Non-keratinised stratified squamous epithelium.	Para-/ortho-keratinised epithelium with extensive infolding. Can be chronically inflamed and resemble radicular cyst lining.

Contents	Degenerating epithelial and inflammatory cells; serum proteins with raised Ig levels; water and electrolytes; cholesterol crystals.	Autolysing parakeratinised cells; low soluble protein (<3.5g/dl) mainly comprised of albumin.

Explanation 4:
Extract 35 and 36 and enucleate the cystic area. Take a post-operative OPT to make sure there is no pathological fracture and give soft-diet advice to the patient. Review after one week, three months, six months and then 12 months, re-radiographing each time to determine whether or not the area is resolving or there has been recurrence.

Case 32 Dental pain

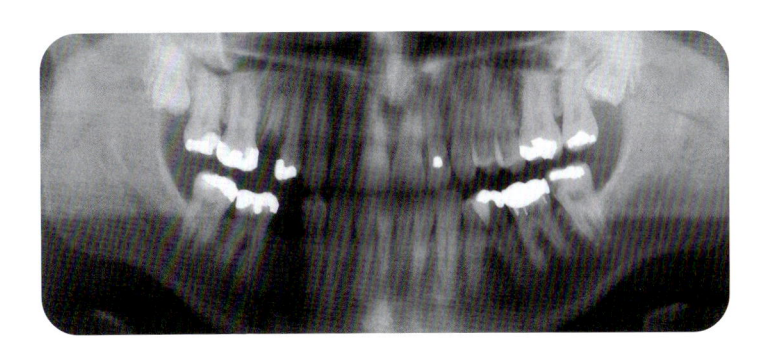

This 35-year-old patient complained of severe intermittent pain on the right side of his mouth that radiated to his right ear and was preventing him from biting on the right side of his mouth. He has hereditary angioedema and is currently taking danazol for this condition. He has no known allergies.

Question 1:
What is the underlying cause of hereditary angioedema?

Question 2:
What are the clinical implications of this condition?

Question 3:
On examination, 15 is TTP and non-vital. 17 is vital but has subgingival caries deep to the MOL amalgam. From these findings and the OPT, what is the possible cause of his pain?

Question 4:
What is your treatment plan for this patient?

Question 5:
What is disseminated intravascular coagulation?

Explanation 1:
Hereditary angioedema is an inherited C1 esterase inhibitor deficiency; it is inherited as an autosomal dominant trait. Initiating factors include minor trauma, sudden temperature changes and emotional stress, which trigger uncontrolled activation of the classical complement pathway and inhibition of kallikrein, which is required to activate plasminogen. It results in capillary dilatation in the deeper components of the skin and mucosa and an increased tendency to develop intravascular coagulation.[44]

Explanation 2:
As the capillaries dilate they become more permeable, and this leads to the formation of oedema, particularly in the upper respiratory and gastrointestinal tract. In the event of trauma, there is also an increased risk of the development of disseminated intravascular coagulation (DIC). These risks therefore need to be prevented before invasive treatment.

Explanation 3:
The most likely cause for the severe pain this patient is suffering is the broken-down 15 tooth. The pain is characteristic of an acute periapical periodontitis related to a non-vital pulp and an acute periapical abscess.

Explanation 4:
Because of the serious potential complications of any surgical treatment on this patient, any teeth of poor prognosis should be extracted in one appointment with the minimal amount of trauma. To prevent activation of complement a concentrate of C1 esterase inhibitor should be infused before surgery, and fresh frozen plasma should be infused during surgery to prevent disseminated intravascular coagulation (DIC).

Explanation 5:
A pathological process characterised by generalised intravascular activation of haemostasis, resulting in widespread fibrin production and activation of fibrinolysis and consumption of platelets and coagulation factors, leading to significant haemorrhage.

Case 33 Radiographic radio-opacity

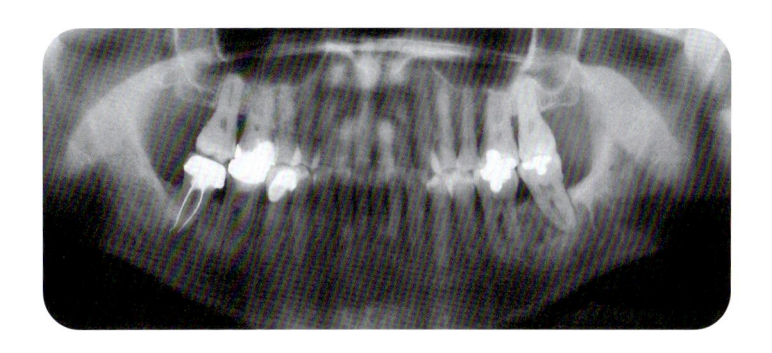

This woman was referred with an unusual incidental radiographic finding on the left side of the mandible. Clinically, there was no history of pain or nerve dysfunction. On examination there was, however, buccolingual bony expansion adjacent to 36 and 37. There was no sinus present and no tenderness on palpation of the area. No teeth were mobile and there was no lymphadenopathy present. Medically, she was fit and not taking any prescribed medication.

Question 1:
Describe the abnormal features on the OPT which the GDP noted.

Question 2:
What is the differential diagnosis for this lesion?

Question 3:
What would you do next in this situation?

Question 4:
How does management of this lesion differ for each possible cause?

Explanation 1:
There is a well circumscribed radio-opaque lesion in the body of the mandible on the left side. It appears to be intimately related to the roots of 36 and 37. The contents appear to be calcified with flecs throughout the mass. There is no resorption of the roots of either tooth.

Explanation 2:
- Benign cementoblastoma.
- Cementifying fibroma.
- Cemental dysplasia.
- Odontogenic fibroma.
- Calcifying epithelial odontogenic tumour (Pindborg tumour).

Explanation 3:
It is imperative that a definitive diagnosis is made, as management of several of these lesions differs substantially. The diagnosis can be made by biopsy of the area in question via an intraoral surgical approach either under local or general anaesthetic.

Explanation 4:
- Benign cementoblastoma: associated tooth extraction.
- Cementifying fibroma: enucleation of the area with extraction of associated teeth.
- Cemental dysplasia: monitor radiographically.
- Odontogenic fibroma: excise lesion and extract related teeth.
- Pindborg tumour: excision of area or local block excision.

Case 34 Lump on tongue

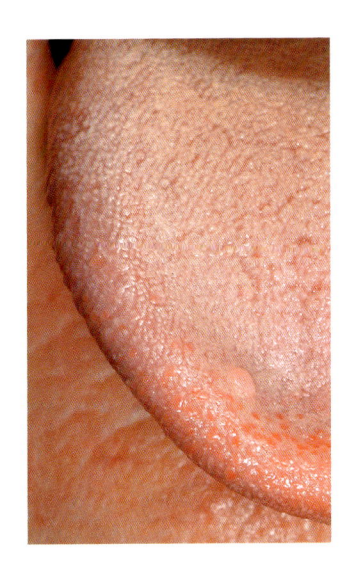

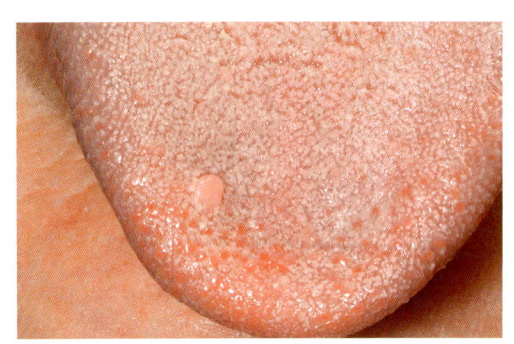

This 54-year-old woman complained of an eight-month history of a painless lump on her tongue. She stated that it had not grown or altered in appearance but that it was annoying her. She was medically fit and well and not taking any prescribed medication. She had no known allergies.

Question 1:
Describe the lesion in the photograph.

Question 2:
From its clinical appearance what do you think it is?

Question 3:
How can this lesion be managed?

Question 4:
In addition, this patient is complaining of a dry mouth. What are the known causes of dry mouth?

Explanation 1:
The photograph shows an exophytic, possibly pedunculated lesion on the dorsum of the tongue. It is the same colour as surrounding tissue and is not ulcerated. There are no rolled margins and no surrounding erythema. It measures approximately 2mm in diameter. The rest of the dorsum of the tongue appears to be normal.

Explanation 2:
There are two possible differential diagnoses for a lesion of this appearance:
- Fibroepithelial polyp.
- Papilloma.

Explanation 3:
As this does not have any features of a malignant lesion, the best way to manage it in view of the irritation it is causing to the patient is to excise it entirely and close the defect primarily with sutures. As a precaution the excised specimen should then be sent for pathological analysis.

Explanation 4:
Dry mouth, or xerostomia, has multiple potential causes:
- Dehydration.
- Mouth-breathing.
- Anxiety.
- Medication (β-blockers and other antihypertensives; antidepressants; psychotropics; antihistamines).
- Sjögren's syndrome.
- Radiotherapy.
- Salivary gland aplasia.
- Ductal atresia.
- HIV-related salivary disease.

Case 35 Facial trauma

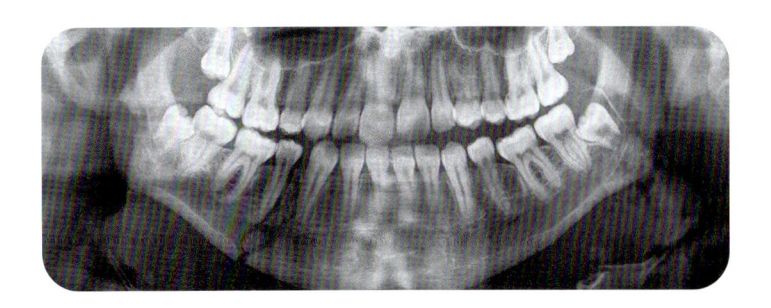

This 18-year-old patient presented following an alleged assault in a nightclub. He was unable to bite together normally and had limitation in opening his mouth. He was otherwise fit and well and not taking any medication. He had no known allergies.

Question 1:
What abnormal features do his radiographs show?

Question 2:
What treatment is required for this?

Question 3:
What information do you need to give this patient in order to obtain informed consent from him?

Question 4:
What advice should you give to this patient before discharging him home?

Explanation 1:
The OPT view shows bilateral fractures to the mandible. On the right side there is a comminuted parasymphyseal fracture and on the left side there is a simple fracture through the angle which appears to traverse the socket of the unerupted third molar on that side. Both fractures are displaced. There do not appear to be any teeth missing, and both condyles appear intact, although a PA X-ray of the jaws is required for confirmation.

Explanation 2:
Because both fractures are displaced and the right-side angle fracture is communicating with the socket of a tooth, the fractures should be repaired surgically via open reduction and internal fixation, using titanium fracture plates. The angle fracture would be easiest accessed transbuccally, and the parasymphyseal fracture can be treated via an intraoral approach.

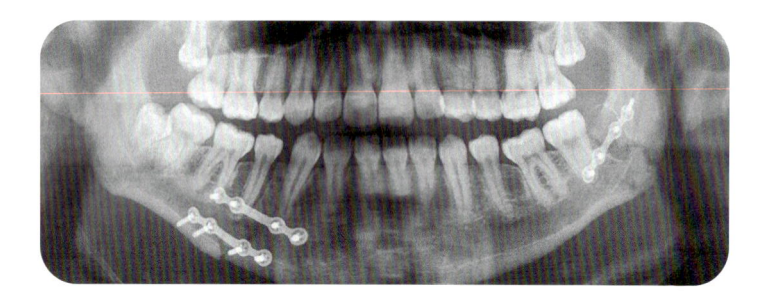

Explanation 3:
- A detailed explanation of his injuries and their location and why they need treating.
- An explanation of the techniques used to repair the fractures, including routes of access (for instance, transbuccal, intraoral) and any teeth that may need to be extracted – 38 in this case.
- The implications of not treating the fractures.
- The risks associated with the surgery (inferior alveolar nerve, mental nerve, lingual nerve damage. Post-operative scarring related to transbuccal approach), post-operative infection, malocclusion.
- What to expect post-operatively (pain, swelling, bruising, sutures intraorally and extraorally).
- All of this should be clearly annotated on a consent form that should be signed and dated by both the patient and surgeon.

Explanation 4:
- Eat a soft diet for six to eight weeks.
- Oral hygiene instruction.
- Analgesia.
- Do not smoke or drink copious alcohol.
- No contact sport for eight weeks.
- Complete a one-week course of broad-spectrum antibiotics.

Case 36 Oral ulcers

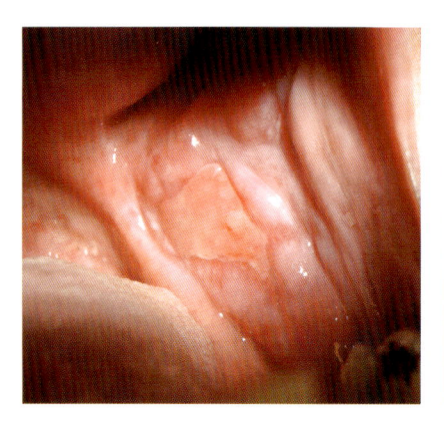

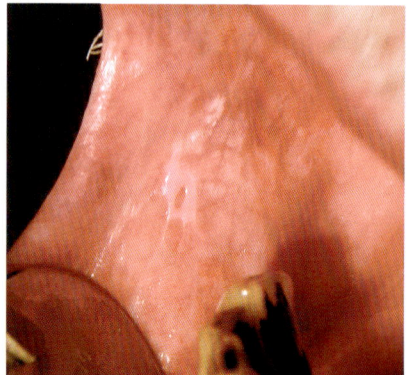

This 85-year-old man complained of a 12-month history of sore mouth and ulcers on his lips and inside his mouth. His medical history is marked by asthma, eczema, acne rosacea and a CVA 15 years ago. He is currently taking aspirin, dipyridamole, clonidine HCl, nabumetone, beclomethasome inhaler, co-dydromol and gabapentin.

Question 1:
What features of note can you see in the photographs?

Question 2:
What tests are required in addition to the clinical examination?

Question 3:
A definitive diagnosis is made of erosive lichen planus. What are the clinical manifestations of this condition?

Question 4:
How would you treat erosive lichen planus?

Explanation 1:
There is a shallow ulcer on the buccal mucosa which has a homogenous base and no rolled margins. There is also a white patch on the opposing buccal mucosa, with surrounding white striae. The patches appear to be homogenous in colour with no sign of interspersed erythema.

Explanation 2:
Because there is ulceration, a full blood count and film should be carried out to ascertain whether there is any underlying haematological problem e.g. anaemia. Because the areas are painful, imprints and rinses should be carried out to see if there is candidal infection present. It may also be desirable to biopsy the area to get a formal diagnosis.

Explanation 3:
Lichen planus is a mucocutaneous disorder that results in lesions of mucosa and skin:
- Purple, pruritic, polygonal papules with or without Wickham's striae on flexor surfaces of the wrists, genital skin, abdominal skin, lumbar regions and neck.
- Alopecia can be a feature.
- Intraorally bilateral white patches with erosions or bullae. There are often surrounding white striae.

Explanation 4:
First ascertain whether or not there is an identifiable cause for the lesions – for instance, drugs (tetracyclines, streptomycin, NSAIDS, sulphonylureas, thiazide diuretics, ACE inhibitors, gold, penicillamine, antimalarials) or associated systemic disease (primary biliary cirrhosis, chronic active hepatitis, graft-versus-host disease, hepatitis C). Medication may be changed, and disease may be treated or stabilised. If not, treat with beclomethasone dipropionate mouthwashes plus or minus intralesional triamcinolone.

Case 37 Oral cancer treatment

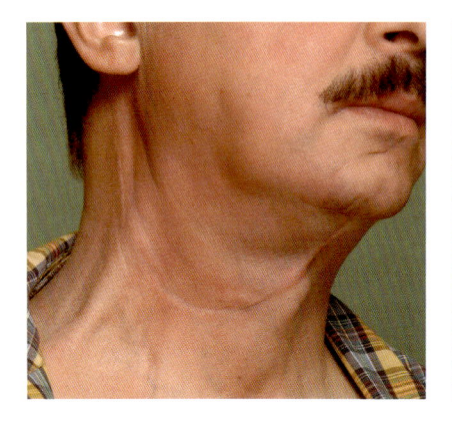

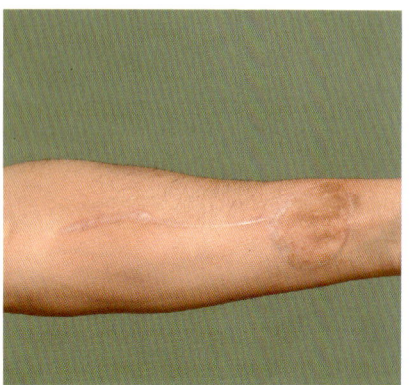

This 45-year-old patient presented for a review appointment at a maxillofacial clinic.

Question 1:
What are these photographs showing?

Question 2:
What are the principles of dental management in patients before radiotherapy?

Question 3:
What are the effects of radiation on the oral tissues?

Part I – Case 37

Explanation 1:
The photograph shows the neck of a male Caucasian patient. There is a scar extending from the inferior border of the chin to the mastoid region on the right side. This scar appears to be following the skin creases of the neck and is the line of incision for a neck dissection. The photograph of the forearm is showing a healed full-thickness graft site following the raising of a radial forearm free flap, which is shown in its new site in the right tonsillar region in the third photograph. This patient has received surgery for a cancer of the right tonsillar region, which involved neck dissection, tonsillar excision and a radial forearm free flap reconstruction.

Explanation 2:
- Perform a thorough oral examination of the patient and assess for treatment need.
- Perform any surgical treatment that is likely to be a problem after radiotherapy.
- Control caries and instruct the patient in prevention:
    - Carry out full mouth scaling.
    - Give oral hygiene instruction.
    - Prescribe daily fluoride mouthwash (0.05% NaF).
    - Regular follow-up.
- Restore all restorable teeth.
- Assess any prosthesis to prevent postradiation trauma from ill-fitting dentures.[17]

Explanation 3:
Three principal pathological states arise in tissues as a sequelae of radiotherapy;[18] these are:
- Hypovascularity.
- Hypoxia.
- Hypocellularity.

The effects of these on the individual oral tissues is as follows:
- *Bone* – decreased vascularity and cellular damage resulting in poor healing following trauma and an increased risk of osteoradionecrosis.

- *Teeth and periodontal tissues* – cellular damage of the periodontal tissues, making the gingivae friable. Altered oral flora combined with dentine dehydration and enamel loss especially in the radiation field increase the susceptibility to the development of radiation caries. This is further exacerbated by xerostomia.
- *Mucosa* – decreased keratinisation, decreased vascularity, ulceration.

PART II

Questions and answers

The second part of the book presents a selection of cases that focus on restorative dentistry. This is an area that students find difficult and the cases have been selected to provide indications as to how the problems should be approached.

Question 1 Implant options in the edentulous patient

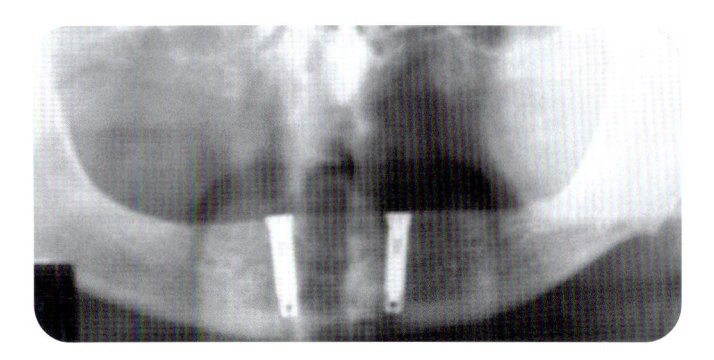

In the edentulous jaws implants can be used to overcome some of the problems of full dentures. Once implants have successfully integrated full arch reconstruction can be completed using either fixed bridges or overdentures.

Question 1:
What is the minimum number of implants usually recommended for (i) fixed bridges and (ii) overdentures in the mandible and maxilla?

Question 2:
The radiograph shows two successfully integrated implants in the mandible. What could be placed on these implants to support an implant-retained overdenture?

Question 3:
Traditional protocols for implants have a healing phase to allow for osseointegration. How long is this in the mandible and the maxilla?

Question 4:
Early loading during the initial healing phase is not recommended as this can lead to movement of the implant within the bone and failure to integrate. What process can occur to prevent successful osseointergration?

Answer 1:
i) Fixed bridges – It is recommended that at least six implants are placed in the edentulous maxilla and four in the edentulous mandible for implant-supported bridges.

ii) Overdentures – It is recommended that four implants are placed in the edentulous maxilla and a minimum of two implants in the edentulous mandible for the support of overdentures.

Answer 2:
The two implants in the mandible could be used to support an implant-retained overdenture with either:
- A gold bar.
- Magnets.
- Ball-ended abutments.

Answer 3:
Following the traditional protocol the healing phase to allow for osseointegration is six months in the maxilla and three months in the mandible.

Answer 4:
Early loading of implants can lead to implants failing to osseointegrate. The loading can cause movement of the implant, and instead of osseointegration a fibrous layer can form between the implant and the bone.

Question 2 Resin-retained bridgework

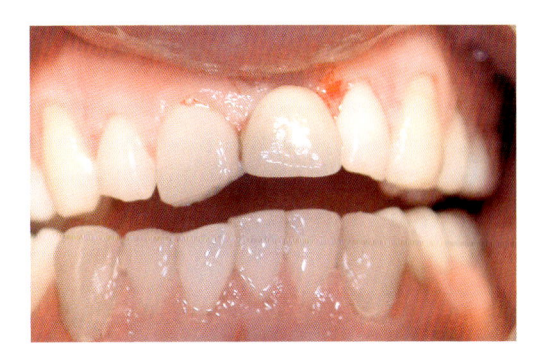

The photograph shows a cantilever resin-retained bridge (RRB) replacing an upper left central.

Question 1:
Why do fixed-fixed RRBs have a higher failure rate than cantilever versions?

Question 2:
Rank in descending order the success of RRBs for the following parts of the mouth:
1. Anterior maxilla
2. Posterior maxilla
3. Anterior mandible
4. Posterior mandible

Question 3:
Name two reasons to explain your least successful choice.

Question 4:
Name one advantage of RRBs over conventional bridges.

Question 5:
Name two disadvantages of RRBs over conventional bridges.

Answer 1:
Fixed-fixed resin-retained bridges have a higher failure rate owing to the differential tooth movement of the retainers, usually causing one wing to debond. This is due to variations in periodontal support, occlusal load and tooth coverage of the two retainers.

Answer 2:
The success rate of RRBs for different areas of the mouth is as follows:
Anterior mandible > anterior maxilla > posterior maxilla > posterior mandible.

Answer 3:
The reasons for a lower success rate in the posterior mandible include:
- Difficult isolation.
- Lingual surface area for bonding is small due to lingual angulation of molars.
- Occlusal factors.

Answer 4:
Advantages of RRBs over conventional bridges include:
- RRB preparations are usually minimal and therefore conservative of tooth structure.
- Cheaper.
- No temporisation of the retainers required.
- Simple impression as margins are supragingival.

Answer 5:
Disadvantages of RRBs over conventional bridges include:
- Cementation is more technique-sensitive, requiring very good isolation.
- Aesthetics can be a problem. This is particularly true with retainers with translucent enamel. The metal wing can often produce shine through greying the incisal third of the tooth.
- Not suitable for large spans.
- Require sound abutment teeth.

Question 3 Implant aesthetics

The radiograph shows an implant placed to restore a missing upper right central incisor.

Question 1:
When a healing abutment is placed after second-stage surgery, how long is it normally left for to allow the soft tissues to mature before an impression is taken for the final crown?

Question 2:
Where should the head of the implant lie in relation to the adjacent teeth to allow for a good emergence profile for the crown?

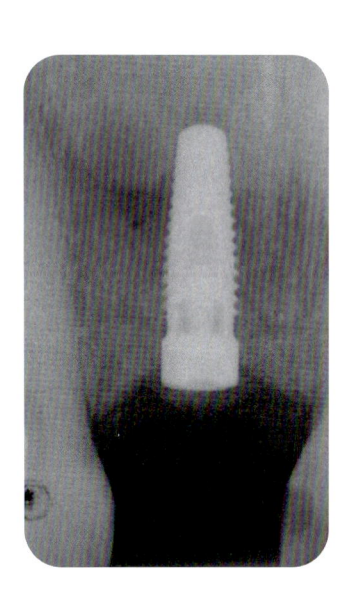

Question 3:
Prior to this implant placement a bone graft procedure was carried out because there was not sufficient bony width in the site for implant placement. Name two intra-oral sites where bone is commonly harvested.

Question 4:
What warnings should be given to the patient with regards to taking bone from the two sites given in your previous answers?

Question 5:
How long between bone grafting and implant placement?

Question 6:
When there is sufficient bone for implant placement but there is a labial concavity present, an alternative grafting procedure can be carried out to improve the aesthetics. Name another type of intra-oral graft procedure that could be used to improve the aesthetics in this region and where it is normally harvested.

Answer 1:
A healing abutment is usually left in place for 3-4 weeks to allow the soft tissues to mature.

Answer 2:
To allow for the implant crown to emerge from the gingiva the implant should be placed so that there will be 2-3mm of gingival tissue above the implant head. To attain this, the implant should be placed 2-3mm apical to the cervical gingival margin of the adjacent teeth.

Answer 3:
Intra-oral bone grafts for small bony defects are commonly taken from the chin region below the apices of the lower incisors or from the ramus of the mandible.

Answer 4:
The patient should be warned that they will develop pain and swelling from either procedure and possible trismus following removal of bone from the ramus. They should also be warned of the risk to the vitality of the lower centrals if bone is taken from the chin.

Answer 5:
Following a bone-grafting procedure it is normally left for a period of three months before implants are placed. If it is left too long there is a risk that the bone graft will resorb.

Answer 6:
If there is sufficient bone to place the implant then a connective tissue graft can be used to 'plump out' the tissues to improve the aesthetics. This is usually taken from the palate in the premolar/molar region.

Question 4 Laminate veneer preparations

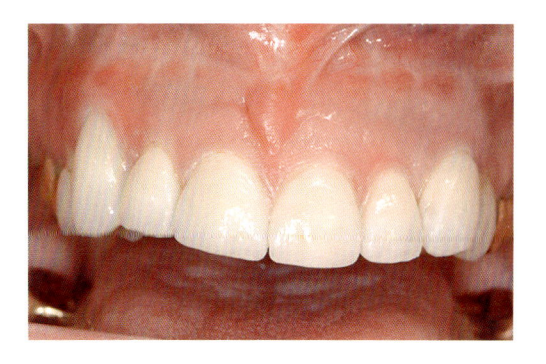

The photograph shows six anterior teeth restored with porcelain veneers.

Question 1:
Describe four different incisal veneer preparations.

Question 2:
It is recommended that, where possible, veneer preparations should be maintained within enamel and follow the contour of the tooth. Describe an ideal veneer preparation with reference to how much enamel you would remove from the cervical, body and incisal area of an upper central incisor to minimise dentine exposure.

Question 3:
Why is it better to have proximal finishing lines that do not extend through the contact points?

Question 4:
What three components make up the final colour of a fitted veneer?

Answer 1:
Veneer preparations can be of the following types:
- Window preparation, where the preparation maintains the incisal edge.
- Feathered preparation, where the preparation ends at the incisal edge with no reduction of the incisal edge, maintaining the palatal aspect of the incisal edge.
- Bevel preparation, where the incisal edge is reduced with no preparation of the palatal surface.
- Incisal overlap preparation, where the incisal edge is reduced and the finishing line is a chamfer finish on the palatal aspect.

Answer 2:
The ideal veneer preparation should be maintained within enamel following the contour of the tooth. This means that the amount of enamel reduction will vary from the cervical margin to the incisal edge. Starting at the gingival margin, the preparation depth will need to be of the order of 0.4mm, gradually rising to 0.7mm, for the bulk of the preparation.

Answer 3:
Wherever possible it is best not to take the veneer preparation through the contact points because without very good temporisation the adjacent teeth may move, preventing seating of the veneer. This may cause the veneer to fracture at the time of cementation.

Answer 4:
The final colour of a veneer restoration is dependent on three factors: the underlying tooth colour, the cement and the veneer itself.

Question 5 Management of the discoloured tooth

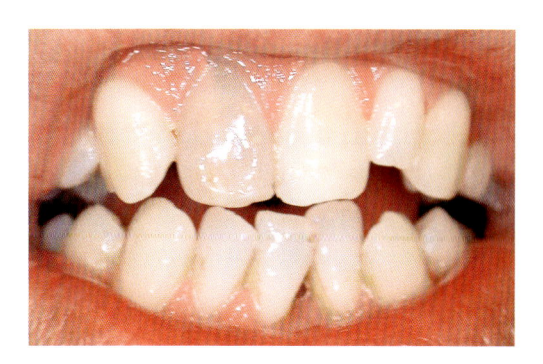

The photograph shows a discoloured upper right central incisor.

Question 1:
What is the likely cause of this discolouration?

Question 2:
Describe the mechanism that has lead to this discolouration.

Question 3:
What three options are available to manage this discolouration?

Question 4:
Outline the advantages and disadvantages of each method.

Answer 1:
This discolouration is caused by loss of pulp vitality, leading to pulpal necrosis. In this case it was associated with trauma.

Answer 2:
The discolouration is caused by one of two things. First, blood degradation products release iron during haemolysis, which can be converted to black ferric sulphide by bacteria. Secondly, the discolouration can be caused by degrading proteins of the necrotic pulp.

Answer 3:
This tooth was root-filled. The discolouration could be managed by either:
- Internal bleaching.
- Veneers.
- Crowns or post crowns.

Answer 4:
Internal bleaching is the least invasive procedure and can be an effective way of dealing with the discolouration. The disadvantages are that, in some cases, the discolouration returns and there is the risk of causing resorption.

Veneers are less destructive than crowns, but it may be difficult to mask the discolouration without heavy preparation or without requiring the use of an opaque cement or a larger amount of opaque porcelain, which may produce lifeless-looking restorations.

Crowns will ultimately provide an aesthetic restoration, but this is the most destructive procedure and if there is little coronal tissue remaining may require post preparations. Post preparations require removal of a large amount of coronal and radicular tooth substance, possibly putting the teeth at risk of root fracture.

Question 6 Non-vital bleaching

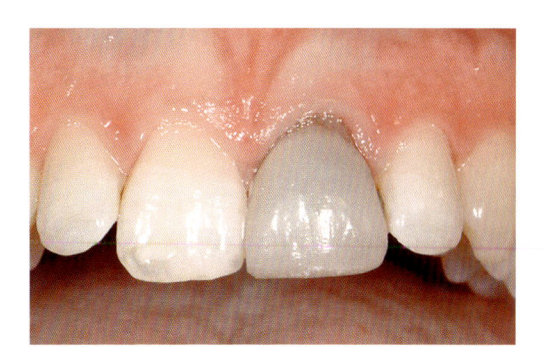

The photograph shows a discoloured tooth that has previously been root-filled and veneered.

Question 1:
Describe the procedure for internal bleaching.

Question 2:
Name three chemicals that can be used in internal bleaching.

Question 3:
What warnings should a patient be given before the start of internal bleaching?

Question 4:
What is the advantage of the application of heat to the process of internal bleaching and what is its disadvantage?

Question 5:
Other than pulp necrosis what else can cause tooth discolouration?

Answer 1:
The procedure for internal bleaching involves the following:
- The tooth is isolated, preferably with a rubber dam.
- The restoration in the access cavity is completely removed.
- The coronal root filling material is removed to below the cemento-enamel junction. This can be confirmed with the use of a Williams periodontal probe.
- The removal should be sufficient to allow for a base to be placed over the root-filling material (usually Poly-F).
- The bleaching material is placed in the access cavity (heat or light may be applied).
- The material is sealed in the tooth with a temporary restorative material.
- The tooth is reviewed one to two weeks later and the procedure is repeated, if necessary.

Answer 2:
Hydrogen peroxide alone or in conjunction with sodium perborate may be used as the bleaching agent. The alternatives are sodium perborate mixed with water or carbamide peroxide.

Answer 3:
- The patient should be warned of the risk of external cervical resorbtion.
- The treatment may take 2-3 visits and if treatment has not produced the desired results after three attempts, further changes in colour will be minimal.
- If the discolouration is caused by restoration materials such as amalgam, then treatment may not be successful.

Answer 4:
The application of heat to accelerate the process of internal bleaching is not recommended because of its association with external cervical resorbtion.

Answer 5:
Coronal discolouration is not always caused by necrotic pulps. Restorative materials such as amalgams can also cause discolouration. Root-filling materials can also cause discolouration, as can intra-canal medicaments such as Ledermix.

Question 7 Gingival recession and periodontal splints

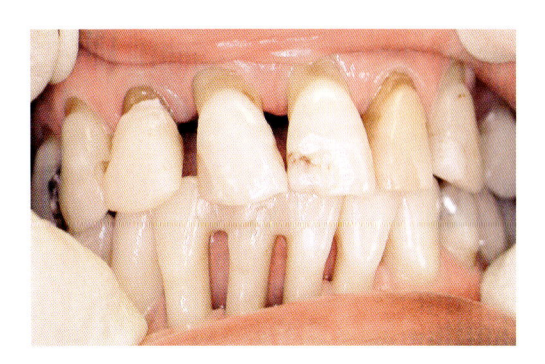

The photograph shows a patient with periodontal disease.

Question 1:
The maxillary dentition shows marked gingival recession. List five causative factors that could be associated with this process.

Question 2:
The lower anterior teeth have been splinted. What benefit does this provide to these teeth?

Question 3:
Briefly describe four techniques for periodontal splinting.

Answer 1:
A number of causative factors are associated with gingival recession. These include:
- Periodontal disease.
- Alveolar bone dehiscences.
- Iatrogenic damage (for instance, restorative treatment, periodontal treatment, orthodontic treatment).
- Toothbrush trauma.
- Tooth malposition.
- Traumatic overbite.
- Self-inflicted gingival trauma.
- Drug-related (for instance, cocaine abuse).

Answer 2:
Periodontal splinting of mobile teeth allows improved function of the mobile teeth.

Answer 3:
There are a number of techniques for splinting periodontally involved teeth. These include:
- Direct composite bonded along the lingual surface – but this needs to be rather bulky and is liable to fracture.
- Composite and wire – a twistflex wire can be bent to the shape of the lingual surface on a model of the teeth and then held by smaller amounts of composite intra-orally.
- Fibre-reinforced materials – for instance, Stick-tech, can be bonded to hold mobile teeth.
- Linked crowns.
- Metal retainers, cast and bonded to the lingual surfaces.

Question 8 Management of palatal toothwear

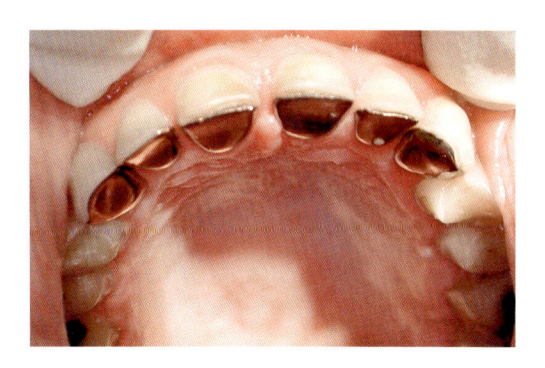

The photograph shows a tooth-wear case restored with gold palatal veneers.

Question 1:
Why is gold a good material for the restoration of the palatal surfaces of these teeth?

Question 2:
What disadvantage is there to using gold?

Question 3:
Non-precious metals can be used for this technique as well. Name three disadvantages of these materials compared with gold.

Question 4:
For gold veneers to be bonded to teeth the fitting surface needs to be treated. One technique produces a stable oxide layer. What percentage of copper content is required to produce this layer?

Question 5:
Name two other techniques used to surface-treat gold veneers.

Question 6:
What alternative materials could be used to restore the palatal surfaces?

Answer 1:
Gold is a good material to use for the restoration of the palatal surfaces of these teeth because it is easy to adjust and is not abrasive to the apposing dentition.

Answer 2:
The disadvantage of using gold (or any other metal) for the management of tooth wear cases is that you can get shine-through that can give a grey appearance to the incisal third of the tooth.

Answer 3:
Non-precious metals have also been used for the management of palatal tooth wear. The disadvantages of non-precious metals are:
- Non-precious metal castings are not as accurate as gold castings.
- They are very hard materials and therefore more difficult to adjust and re-polish.
- They are more abrasive and therefore can cause more damage to the opposing dentition.

Answer 4:
The copper content of gold veneers needs to be greater than 7% to create an appropriate oxide layer for bonding.

Answer 5:
Three other techniques can be used to treat the fitting surface of gold.
- Silicoter – silicon oxides are deposited onto the surface of the gold.
- Tin-plating – produces a stable oxide layer.
- Sandblasting of the metal surface.

Answer 6:
Apart from gold or non-precious metals composite or porcelain can be used.

Question 9 Management of gingival recession

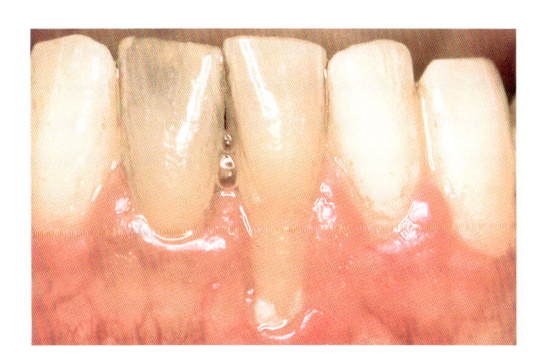

The photograph shows an area of gingival recession affecting a lower central incisor.

Question 1:
What are the indications for the treatment of gingival recession?

Question 2:
This area can be managed with either a free gingival graft or a connective tissue graft. The donor site is commonly taken from the palate. Which region of the palate is usually used for the donor site?

Question 3:
Which anatomical structures need to be avoided to prevent complications?

Question 4:
Name two other surgical procedures that can be used to treat gingival recession.

Question 5:
Name three factors that could influence the success of surgery.

Answer 1:
The indications for treating gingival recession include:
- Improvement of aesthetics.
- Prevention of continued recession.
- Sensitivity.
- Management of root caries.

Answer 2:
Palatal grafts are usually taken from the premolar and first molar region.

Answer 3:
It is important to avoid the greater palatine neurovascular bundle.

Answer 4:
In some instances gingivae can be treated with a rotational flap procedure (laterally repositioned flap, oblique rotational flap, double papilla procedure) or with a coronally repositioned flap.

Answer 5:
Factors that may influence the success of surgery include:
- Control of causative factors: these should be identified and addressed before surgery.
- The width of the defect: in larger defects the proportion of avascular tissue donated will be greater and dependent on a larger recipient-site blood supply.
- Whether the patient is a smoker.

Question 10 Partial dentures and free end saddles

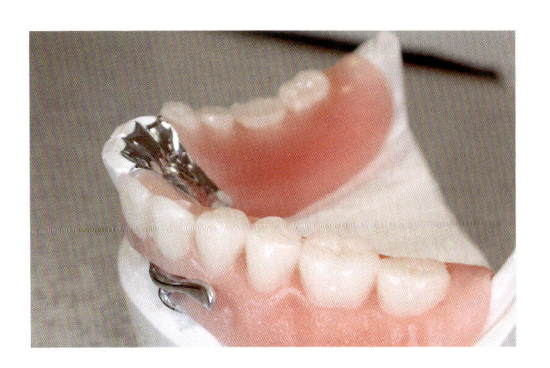

The photograph shows a lower partial denture.

Question 1:
What type of denture is this?

Question 2:
What is the Kennedy classification for this denture?

Question 3:
What patient factors may make this an inappropriate denture design?

Question 4:
For which clinical situation is this type of denture usually indicated?

Question 5:
What are the advantages of this type of denture design?

Question 6:
What should be considered before deciding which side the hinge should be placed?

125

Answer 1:
The photograph shows a swinglock lower denture.

Answer 2:
The Kennedy classification for this denture is Class I.

Answer 3:
Patients with poor manual dexterity may find this type of denture difficult to use. It would be inappropriate to prescribe this type of denture to patients with poor oral hygiene. Its design covers a large area of gingivae, both labially and lingually. Plaque accumulation under such a denture could quickly lead to caries and gingival problems.

Answer 4:
This type of denture is traditionally used for lower bilateral free end saddle cases where only the anterior teeth remain. These teeth often have insufficient undercuts for conventional clasping. It can also get around the problem of unsightly clasping units, which some patients find unacceptable.

Answer 5:
The advantages of this type of denture include:
- Avoidance of unacceptable clasping units.
- The addition of the acrylic veneer onto the swinging labial bar can improve aesthetics in patients with gingival recession and a low lip line.
- Improved retention and stability.

Answer 6:
Before deciding on which side to place the hinge it is worth finding out if the patient is left or right-handed so it can be placed on the side that is easiest to secure and remove.

Question 11 Management of the perio-endo lesion

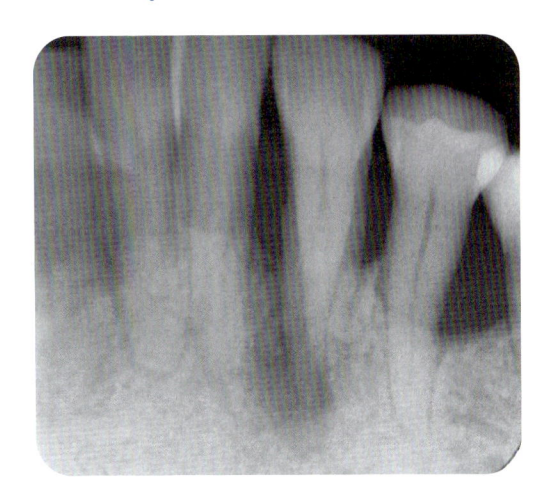

The X-ray shows a radiograph of a two-rooted lower left canine that has a perio-endo lesion.

Question 1:
Name five ways in which communication can occur between the periodontium and the pulp.

Question 2:
What investigations need to be carried out before treating suspected perio-endo lesions?

Question 3:
Which treatment should usually be carried out first – endodontic or periodontal – in the management of perio-endo lesions?

Question 4:
What is the rationale behind this?

Clinical Short-Answer Questions For Postgraduate Dentistry

Answer 1:
Communication can occur between the pulp and the periodontium via the following ways:
- The apical foramen.
- Dentine tubules.
- Lateral root canals.
- Furcation root canals.
- Root fractures.

Answer 2:
Before treating suspected perio-endo lesions it is important to vitality-test the tooth and carry out a periodontal examination with a probe.

Answer 3:
If a perio-endo lesion is present it is normal to start with endodontic treatment first.

Answer 4:
The rationale behind this is that periodontal lesions sometimes resolve following successful endodontic treatment. This is never true of the reverse. When there is a true perio-endo lesion periodontal treatment alone may lead to initial healing, but in the presence of pulpal infection this will rapidly breakdown.

Question 12 Tooth discolouration

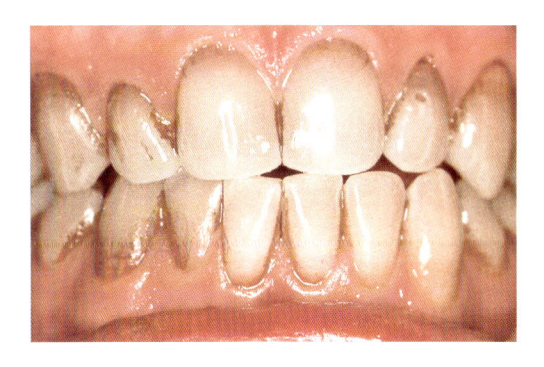

The photograph shows dental staining caused by a mouthwash.

Question 1:
Name the chemical that has caused the discolouration.

Question 2:
What other oral side-effects have been reported with the use of products containing this chemical?

Question 3:
Describe why staining occurs with this product.

Question 4:
What are the modes of action of this mouthwash?

Answer 1:
Chlorhexidine is the chemical that has caused this staining.

Answer 2:
This chemical is also associated with oral side-effects, which include:
- Altered taste sensation.
- Unpleasant taste.
- Increased supragingival calculus formation.
- Unilateral or bilateral parotid swellings.
- Staining of the dorsum of the tongue.
- Mucosal erosions.
- Mucosal burning sensations.

Answer 3:
Staining occurs with this chemical because it adsorbs to the tooth surface and precipitates dietary chromogens.

Answer 4:
Chlorhexidine has two modes of action: it is both an antiseptic agent and an anti-plaque agent.

Its antiseptic action stems from the fact that it is a dicationic bisguanide, which adsorbs to the negatively charged bacterial cell wall. At low concentrations it is bacteriostatic and at high concentrations it is bactericidal.

Its anti-plaque mode of action is due to its ability to adsorb to receptors within the tooth pellicle, providing a persistent bacteriostatic effect lasting 12-14 hours.

Question 13 Edentulous ridges

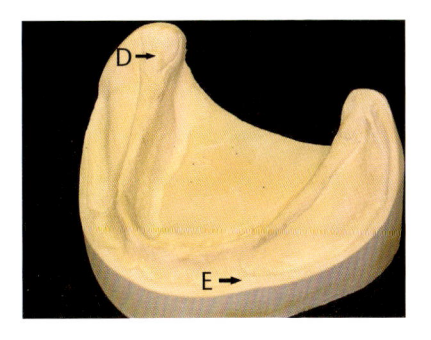

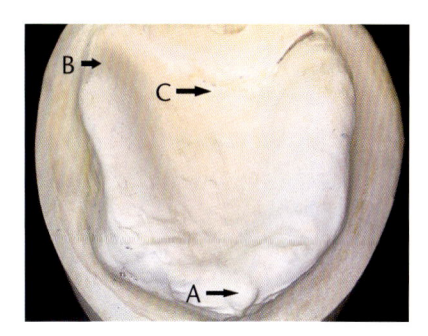

The photographs show maxillary and mandibular edentulous ridges of a patient who recently had new complete upper and lower dentures constructed.

Question 1:
Name the five anatomical landmarks indicated by the arrows A-E.

Question 2:
The patient presented at review complaining that the upper denture dropped during function. Suggest two technical reasons for this problem.

Question 3:
How would you rectify these problems?

Clinical Short-Answer Questions For Postgraduate Dentistry

Answer 1:
The anatomical landmarks are:
- A. Incisive papilla.
- B. Hamular notch.
- C. Fovea palatinus.
- D. Retromolar pad.
- E. Buccal frenum.

Answer 2:
The most common reasons for a well-fitting upper complete denture dropping during function are:
- Over-extension in the buccal sulcus or around the muscle attachments.
- Occlusal interferences with premature contacts.

Answer 3:
If the denture is over-extended these areas need to be identified and reduced.

If there are occlusal interferences these must be identified and adjusted. If the discrepancy is small, these can be adjusted at chairside to give a balanced occlusion.

If there is more than just a small discrepancy, a pre-centric record should be taken and the dentures articulated in the laboratory and adjusted accordingly to give a balanced occlusion. If it is considered a large discrepancy then removing of the posterior teeth and re-recording the occlusion for a new set up may be more appropriate.

Question 14 Gingival enlargement

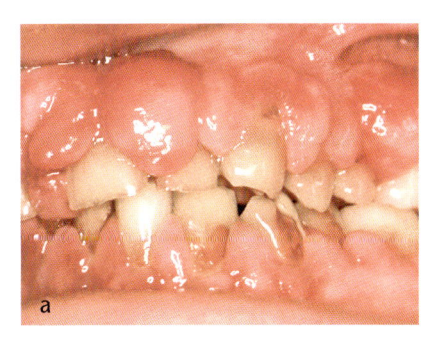

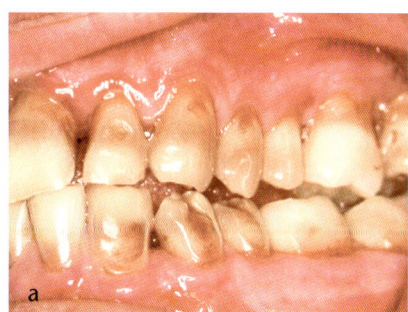

The photographs show (a) pre-operative and (b) post-operative pictures of a patient who has had a renal transplant.

Question 1:
Describe the appearance of the gingiva in (a) and name the procedure that has been carried out to achieve the appearance shown in (b).

Question 2:
Name the immunosupressive agent commonly used by renal transplant patients that is associated with this appearance.

Question 3:
Name an alternative immunosupressive agent which does not cause this gingival condition.

Question 4:
Name two other types of drugs associated with this gingival appearance.

Question 5:
Name the autosomal dominant condition that is associated with generalised gingival enlargement.

Question 6:
Gingival swelling can also associated with Crohn's disease. What other oral manifestations have been noted with this condition?

Answer 1:
The gingivae in (a) appears hyperplastic with gingival overgrowth over part of the maxillary dentition. This condition has been managed with a gingivectomy, shown in (b).

Answer 2:
Cyclosporin is the commonly used immunosuppressive agent that causes the gingival overgrowth.

Answer 3:
Tacrolimus is a relatively new alternative anti-rejection drug that has been shown to have less potential to cause gingival overgrowth in transplant patients (others include sirolimus and mycophenolate mofetil).

Answer 4:
- Anticonvulsants such as phenytoin and sodium valporate.
- Calcium channel blockers such as nifedipine, diltiazem and amlodipine.

Answer 5:
The autosomal dominant condition associated with generalised gingival enlargement is hereditary gingival fibromatosis.

Answer 6:
Crohn's disease can also be associated with gingival enlargement. Some of the other oral conditions associated with this disease include:
- Oral ulceration.
- Thickening and folding of the oral mucosa, producing a 'cobblestone' appearance and mucosal tags.
- Lip swellings, splitting of the lips and angular cheilitis.

Question 15 Fibre posts

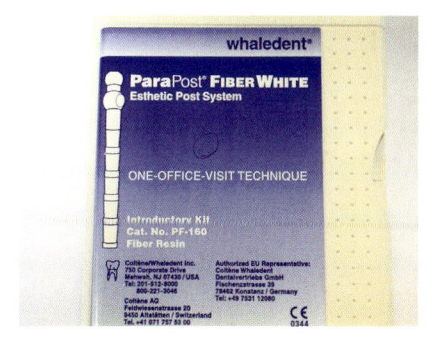

The photograph shows a glass-fibre post system.

Question 1:
What advantage does this system have over a carbon-fibre post system?

Question 2:
Briefly describe the advantages of non-metal post systems compared with metal posts.

Question 3:
What factors predispose to root fracture with post restorations?

Question 4:
What is a ferrule and what are the reasons for using one?

Answer 1:
Carbon-fibre posts are black in colour and so can affect the aesthetic result when ceramic crowns are placed. Glass-fibre posts are colourless or white and therefore overcome this problem.

Answer 2:
Non-metal posts are seen to have a number of advantages over metal-post systems. These include:
- Reduced incidence of root fracture with non-metal post systems.
- It is considered that the removal of fibre-post systems is easier than metal post systems.
- Non-metal posts do not undergo corrosion. This can produce better aesthetic results, as corrosion products can pass into the root and discolour it.
- In cases where there is insufficient dentine supragingivally to create a ferrule the bonding of non-fibre posts may reinforce the root.

Answer 3:
Factors that predispose a root to fracture with post restorations include:
- An inadequate thickness of dentine.
- The use of tapered posts.
- The use of threaded posts.
- Short posts.
- Not using a ferrule of adequate length and taper.

Answer 4:
A ferrule is an encircling band of cast metal around the coronal surface of the tooth. The reason for using one is to reinforce root-filled teeth and reduce the chance of root fracture.

Question 16 Painful gums

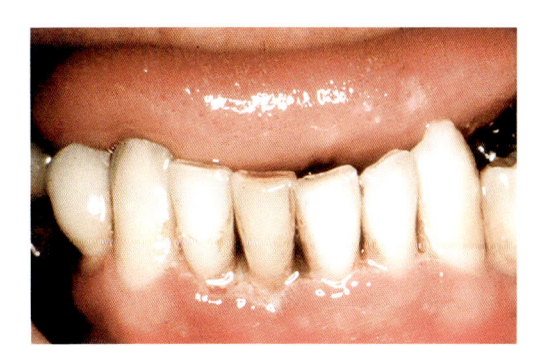

The photograph shows the gingiva of a patient complaining of painful bleeding gums.

Question 1:
What is the likely cause of this condition?

Question 2:
What aetiological factors are associated with this condition?

Question 3:
What micro-organisms are associated with this condition?

Question 4:
Which age group is more commonly affected?

Question 5:
What other group of patients may be affected?

Question 6:
How would you treat this condition?

Answer 1:
The photograph shows a case of necrotic ulcerative gingivitis (NUG).

Answer 2:
NUG is a plaque-induced gingival disease and is predisposed in young patients in their second and third decades. It is has been associated with smoking and emotional stress.

Answer 3:
The species of bacteria associated with this condition, giving rise to a fuso-spirochaetal complex, are:
- Fusobacterium species.
- Spirochaetes.

Answer 4:
NUG is more commonly seen in the second and third decades of life.

Answer 5:
This condition is also seen in immunocompromised groups, such as people with HIV infection.

Answer 6:
This condition is normally treated with oral hygiene instruction, scaling and metronidazole 200 mg three times daily for three days. The use of sodium perborate mouthwash can also be used during the acute phase, when brushing is too painful.

Question 17 Fluorosis

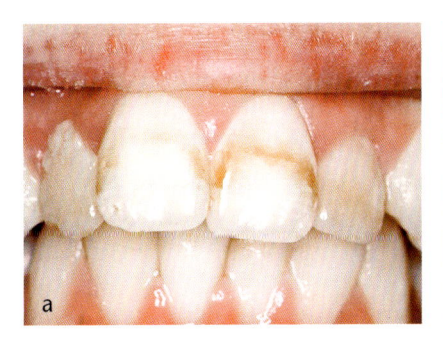

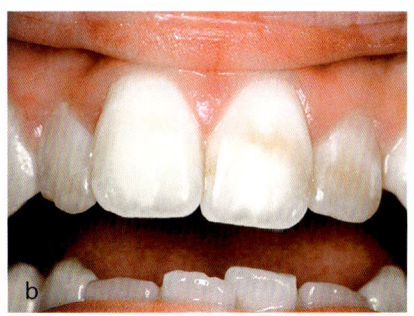

The photographs show anterior teeth (a) before, and (b) after undergoing a procedure.

Question 1:
What procedure has been used here to improve dental appearance?

Question 2:
Fluorosis can produce a very similar appearance to photograph (a). What level of fluoride can lead to fluorosis?

Question 3:
Describe the stages of the procedure used to improve the appearance shown in photograph (b).

Question 4:
Name two clinical situations where this procedure could be indicated as a suitable treatment to improve enamel aesthetics, other than fluorosis.

Question 5:
Name two clinical appearances where it is not recommended.

Answer 1:
The improvement in appearance between (a) and (b) has followed the use of microabrasion.

Answer 2:
Fluorosis is caused during amelogenesis and is associated with fluoride levels of 5 ppm.

Answer 3:
The technique for microabrasion is as follows:
- Clean teeth with pumice and water.
- Isolate with rubber dam and paint copalite around the necks of the dam or apply vaseline under the dam.
- Sodium bicarbonate is mixed with water and applied to the dam behind the teeth.
- A mix of 18% hydrochloric acid and pumice slurry is applied to the tooth and agitated for five to 10 seconds with either a wooden spatula or a slowly rotating rubber cup.
- This can be repeated up to 10 times.
- Fluoride is then applied to the surface for two to three minutes.
- After removal of the rubber dam the teeth are polished, using fluoride toothpaste.

Answer 4:
Apart from the management of fluorosis, microabrasion is indicated for the following:
i) Post-orthodontics for the management of surface decalcification defects.
ii) Idiopathic speckling.
iii) White or brown lesions or surface hypoplasia secondary to trauma or infection of a deciduous predecessor.

Answer 5:
Microabrasion is not recommended for the management of amelogenesis imperfecta, dentinogenesis imperfecta or for tetracycline staining.

Question 18 Crown preparations

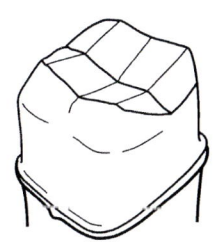

The diagram shows an outline drawing of a crown preparation.

Question 1:
Define retention form and resistance form in relation to a crown preparation.

Question 2:
Which cusp requires a functional cusp bevel on:
  i) A mandibular first molar?
  ii) A maxillary first molar?

Question 3:
What is the reason for the functional cusp bevel?

Question 4:
What is the ideal taper of a porcelain-fused-to-metal crown preparation?

Question 5:
Describe the four features of a crown preparation that will provide resistance to crown removal.

Clinical Short-Answer Questions For Postgraduate Dentistry

Answer 1:
- Retention form prevents removal of the restoration in the long axis of the tooth.
- Resistance form is defined as those features of the preparation that prevent dislodgement of the restoration by forces other than those seeking to remove it in the long axis.

Answer 2:
- The functional cusp of a mandibular molar is the buccal cusp.
- The functional cusp of a maxillary molar is the palatal cusp.

Answer 3:
The reason for the placement of a functional cusp bevel is to increase the bulk of material over the functional cusp to improve structural durability.

Answer 4:
The optimum taper of a preparation is between five to 10 degrees.

Answer 5:
The features of a crown preparation that will provide resistance include:
- The height of the preparation. An increase in height improves resistance.
- The diameter of the preparation.
- The taper.
- The surface texture.

Question 19 Complex denture cases

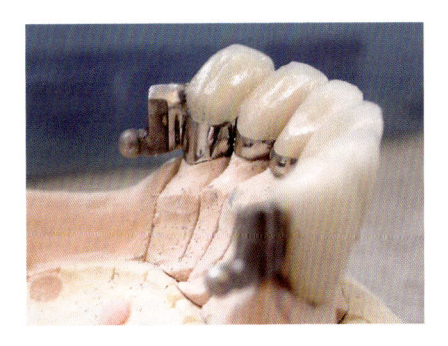

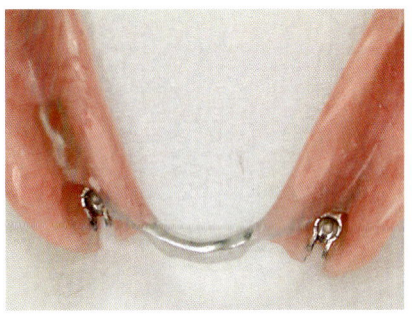

The photographs show the completed laboratory work for a patient, which is to be fitted at her next appointment.

Question 1:
What is the Kennedy classification of this patient's lower arch?

Question 2:
What sort of denture set-up is illustrated?

Question 3:
Name two other clinical situations where attachments can be used.

Question 4:
What are the advantages of this type of denture?

Question 5:
What are the disadvantages?

Answer 1:
The Kennedy classification of this patient is Kennedy Class I.

Answer 2:
This is a precision attachment denture set up with mini-dalbos being used to retain this bilateral free-end denture.

Answer 3:
Precision attachment can be used in a number of clinical situations. These include:
- Overcoming alignment problems where abutments have differing paths of withdrawal.
- Connectors in fixed partial dentures.
- For the retention of overdentures.

Answer 4:
The advantages of this type of denture include:
- Increased retention.
- Increased stability.
- No visible clasping units.

Answer 5:
The disadvantages of this type of denture include:
- More expensive.
- Technically more difficult.
- Good oral hygiene is needed to clean below the attachments and between the linked crowns, requiring a greater level of dexterity on behalf of the patient.
- Greater level of maintenance.

Question 20 Root-canal treatment

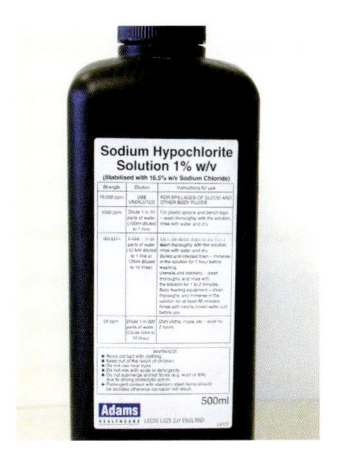

The photograph shows a bottle of sodium hypochlorite, a recommended irrigant for the cleaning of root canals.

Question 1:
Describe three of its properties that make it a useful product?

Question 2:
The use of EDTA is also recommended during the cleaning phase of endodontics. What are the two functions of EDTA in root-canal treatment?

Question 3:
Calcium hydroxide is currently considered the medicament of choice as an intra-canal dressing between appointments. Describe two properties of calcium hydroxide that make it an ideal choice.

Question 4:
Name the bacterial species that can be found in root canals that appear to be resistant to calcium hydroxide.

Question 5:
Name two other antibacterial agents that can be used as an intra-canal medicament between appointments.

Answer 1:
Sodium hypochlorite is a recommended irrigant for the cleaning phase of endodontic treatment. The properties that make this a useful agent include:
- Bactericidal.
- Dissolves organic material.
- Lubricating action.
- Flushing out of debris.
- Bleaches the tooth, reducing staining.

Answer 2:
EDTA has a number of functions: first, it can remove the smear layer and, secondly, it acts as a lubricant.

Answer 3:
Calcium hydroxide is currently considered the medicament of choice due to its antimicrobial effects. It has a high pH value of 12.5, which has destructive effects on cell membranes and protein structures. This antimicrobial effect is due to its ability to release hydroxyl ions. It also has tissue-dissolving properties. When applied correctly in paste format it also acts as a physical barrier to prevent reinfection of the canal.

Answer 4:
Enterococcus faecalis is frequently found in retreatment cases and is resistant to the effects of calcium hydroxide.

Answer 5:
Other dressings used as an intra-canal medicament between appointments include Ledermix, chlorehexidine in gel or preformed point form or 1% parachlorophenol.

Question 21 Infective endocarditis and restorative dentistry

The OPT shows a female patient with advanced chronic adult periodontitis who requires extractions and root surface debridement as part of her treatment, which will be completed under local anaesthetic.

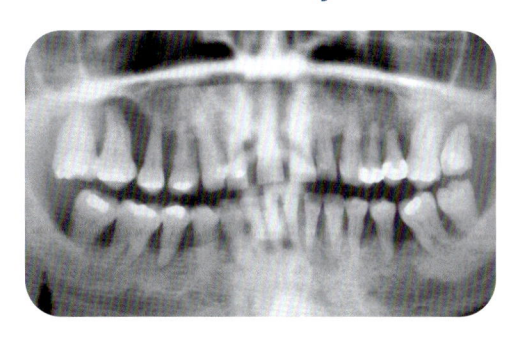

Question 1:
This patient has had previous infective endocarditis and therefore requires antibiotic prophylaxis. She is not allergic to penicillin. What prophylactic regime does she require?

Question 2:
If she was allergic to penicillin what regime could you use?

Question 3:
Which of the following procedures do not require antibiotic prophylaxis?
- Dental extractions.
- Removal of sutures.
- Placement of rubber dam.
- Subgingival placement of antibiotic fibres.
- Intraligamentary local anaesthetic injections.
- Placement of orthodontic brackets.

Question 4:
Which of the following medical conditions require antibiotic prophylaxis?
- Coronary by-pass surgery.
- Ventricular septal defects.
- Cerebrospinal shunts.
- Pacemakers.
- Renal transplant.
- Hypertrophic cardiomyopathy.

Question 5:
Doxycycline has been used as an adjunct for the management of periodontal disease. What should be warned about before taking these tablets?

Answer 1:
The current regime for high-risk patients who need prophylactic cover before specific dental procedures but are not allergic to penicillin is:
- Amoxicillin 1 g IV plus gentamycin 120 mg IV pre-op plus 500 mg amoxicillin orally six hours post-op.

Answer 2:
If the patient is allergic to penicillin a number of different recommended regimes are available, namely:
- Teicoplanin (400 mg) IV plus gentamycin (120 mg) IV pre-op.
- Clindamycin (300 mg) IV given over 10 mins in 50 ml of diluent pre-op plus 150 mg clindamycin six hours later.
- Vancomycin 1g slow IV infusion (not less than 100 mins), followed by gentomycin (120 mg) IV pre-op.

Answer 3:
Prophylaxis is not recommended for the following dental procedures:
- Removal of sutures.
- Placement of rubber dam.
- Placement of orthodontic brackets.

Answer 4:
The following medical conditions require antibiotic prophylaxis:
- Ventricular septal defects.
- Cerebrospinal shunts.
- Hypertrophic cardiomyopathy.

Answer 5:
Patients prescribed doxycycline should be warned of the following side-effects:
- Nausea.
- Photosensitivity.
- Headaches.
- Intracranial hypertension – patients should be warned that if they develop headaches and ocular effects such as diplopia (double vision) they should stop the medication immediately.

Question 22 Designing dentures

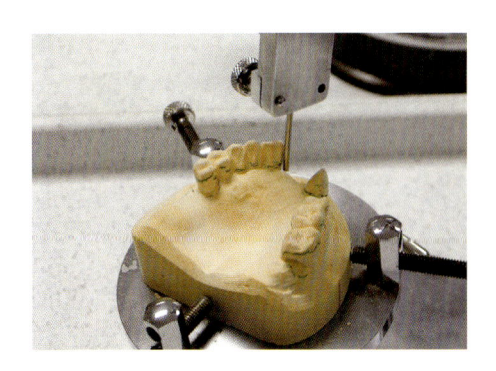

Question 1:
What procedure is demonstrated in the photograph and what component is being used with this piece of equipment?

Question 2:
What are the objectives of this procedure in partial denture design?

Question 3:
In a Kennedy Class I situation where the last tooth in front of each saddle is a premolar, the apparatus is placed on an anterior tilt. Why is this?

Question 4:
What is the minimum depth of functional lingual sulcus required for a lingual bar?

Question 5:
Place the following in the order you should follow when designing a partial denture? Support, retention, saddles, indirect retention, reciprocation and bracing, connectors.

Answer 1:
- The picture shows an upper cast of a partially dentate patient on a surveyor.
- The piece of equipment being used is the analysing rod to identify undercut areas and to determine the parallelism of surfaces.

Answer 2:
The objectives of surveying study models in partial denture design include:
- Finding the optimum path of insertion.
- Deciding the design, material and position of clasps.

Answer 3:
The reason for using an anterior tilt in Kennedy Class I cases, where the last tooth is a premolar, is because there is often an undercut present. By tilting it forward the denture would be designed to fit into these undercuts, preventing dislodgement in a vertical direction.

Answer 4:
The minimum depth of functional lingual sulcus required for a lingual bar is 8mm.

Answer 5:
When designing a partial denture it is recommended that you plan it in the following order:
1. Saddles.
2. Support.
3. Retention.
4. Bracing and reciprocation.
5. Connectors.
6. Indirect retention.

Question 23 Toothwear and dentures

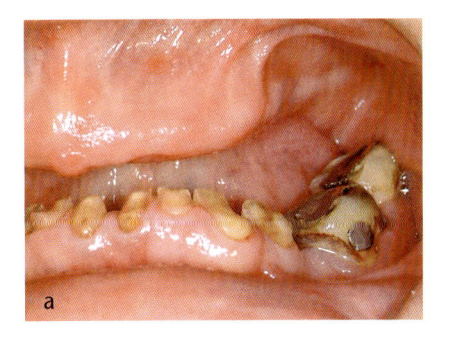

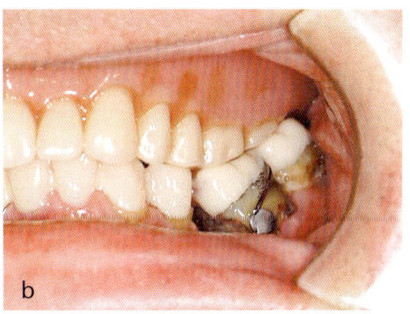

Photograph (a) shows a patient who is edentulous in the maxilla, with advanced tooth wear, affecting his remaining mandibular teeth. Photograph (b) shows the same patient with a complete upper denture and a lower partial denture *in situ*.

Question 1:
What are the differences between:
  i) Overdentures?
  ii) Onlay dentures?
  iii) Overlay dentures?

Question 2:
What are the advantages of maintaining the remaining teeth and constructing either of the three dentures types?

Question 3:
What are the disadvantages of keeping the remaining teeth?

Question 4:
This lower partial denture is a provisional all-acrylic denture. What advantages are there for using a provisional denture in this situation?

Answer 1:
i) Overdentures replace the damaged or missing teeth with prosthetic teeth and an acrylic flange.
ii) Onlay dentures cover only the occlusal or incisal surfaces of the abutment teeth.
iii) Overlay dentures cover the damaged teeth with a full labial veneer facing.

Answer 2:
The advantages of keeping the remaining teeth in either of these types of dentures include:
- Increased support and stability.
- Alveolar bone resorption decreases.
- Improved masticatory efficiency.
- Emotional benefits to the patient.

Answer 3:
The disadvantages are that, owing to the teeth being covered, they are more susceptible to caries and periodontal problems, and therefore maintenance needs can be greater.

Answer 4:
It is considered beneficial to construct a provisional acrylic prosthesis first to allow for modifications in tooth shape position and occlusal relationships to be carried out. It is also perceived to be of benefit to see if the patient can tolerate both the denture and the increase in occlusal vertical dimension (OVD) it creates before going to the final cobalt chrome design. It is not until this point that any tooth preparation should be carried out.

Question 24 Toothwear and composites

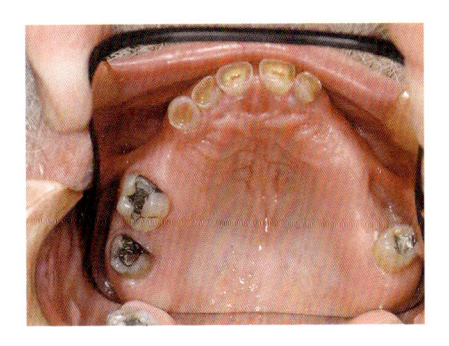

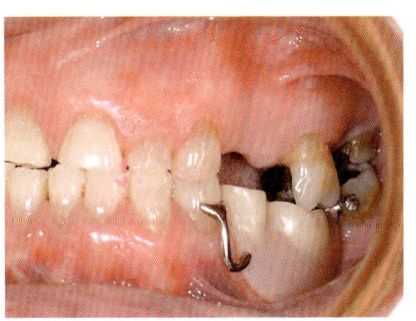

The photographs show a patient with tooth wear affecting his upper anterior teeth.

Question 1:
Describe the appearance and suggest the likely cause.

Question 2:
How should a patient presenting with this appearance be managed initially?

Question 3:
What process has occurred to ensure continuing tooth contact?

Question 4:
The Dahl concept can be used with either a fixed or removable appliance to create anterior space. Describe how the Dahl concept works.

Question 5:
What are the advantages of using composite restorations in cases like this?

Clinical Short-Answer Questions For Postgraduate Dentistry

Answer 1:
The photographs show the patient's remaining anterior teeth with tooth surface loss into dentine, with the pulp canals visible. The dentine has a dished-out appearance with thin enamel margins that show signs of chipping. This is likely to be caused by erosion and attrition.

Answer 2:
Initial management would include:
- Determination of the aetiology and a preventative programme.
- Vitality testing and radiographs.
- Finding out the patient's concerns with this pattern of tooth wear.
- Relieve any sensitivity or pain.

Answer 3:
Maintenance of tooth contact and the occlusal vertical dimension in this case has occurred because of alveolar growth compensating for the wear.

Answer 4:
The Dahl concept creates inter-occlusal space for the placement of anterior restorations in patients with localised tooth-wear. It does this by causing intrusion of the anterior teeth and extrusion or eruption of the posterior teeth.

Answer 5:
The advantages of the use of composite in the management of localised tooth-wear include:
- Simple technique.
- Repairable.
- Easily adjustable.
- Little or no tooth preparation required (conservative).
- Good aesthetics.

Question 25 Dentine bonding

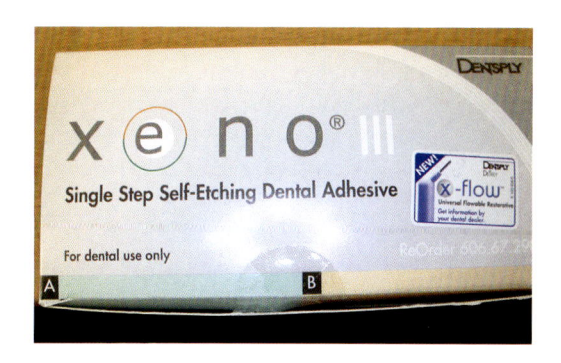

The photograph shows a self-etching dental adhesive.

Question 1:
What is the principle behind wet bonding?

Question 2:
What are the consequences of desiccating dentine following etching?

Question 3:
What are the consequences of over-etching dentine for bonding?

Question 4:
What is the C-factor and how does this relate to the problems of post-operative sensitivity in Class 1 cavities restored with composite?

Question 5:
Dentine is much more difficult to bond to than enamel. Suggest two reasons for this.

Question 6:
What clinical factors may influence the success of dentine bonding?

Answer 1:
The principle behind wet bonding is that, following the etching of dentine, the dentine tubules open up and the collagen fibres stick up, supported by the presence of the water. Keeping the surface of the dentine moist keeps the collagen fibres in an optimum state for infiltration of the primer and adhesive. The primers are carried in a volatile solvent that displaces the water and in the process pull the adhesive into the dentine with them.

Answer 2:
If the dentine is desiccated following the etching stage then the collagen fibres collapse, effectively 'sealing off' the canals from the primer and adhesive. This will lead to an inadequate bond.

Answer 3:
The consequences of over-etching dentine are that resin will not infiltrate to the full depth of demineralisation. This will leave a weak sub-structure, and the bond is likely to fracture.

Answer 4:
The C-Factor is the ratio between bonded surfaces and non-bonded surfaces. The greater the number of bonded surfaces, the greater the C-Factor value. Composite on light curing will contract away from the bonded surfaces. In Class 1 cavities there are five surfaces to pull away from. It is advised that you incrementally pack these cavities in such a way that a minimum number of surfaces is bonded to at once. Reducing the stresses of contraction is less likely to lead to de-bonding and post-operative sensitivity.

Answer 5:
Dentine is considered more difficult to bond to than enamel because:
- A differential pressure exists between the pulp and dentine floor which pumps out fluid, making it impossible to create dry dentine.
- Excess desiccation can cause pulpal damage.
- Dentine is hydrophilic, whereas most adhesives are hydrophobic.
- Dentine is a vital tissue.
- Dentine is covered by a smear layer.

Answer 6:

Clinical factors that may influence the success of bonding to dentine include:
- The age of the patient. Increased sclerotic dentine is more difficult to achieve bonding.
- Tooth position. Maxillary teeth are better than mandibular teeth for bonding.
- The depth of the cavity.
- Contamination of dentine with blood, saliva or oil.

References for Part I

1. Deodhar AK, Rana RE. Surgical physiology of wound healing: a review. J Postgrad Med 1997;43:52-56.
2. Lamey PJ, Darwazeh AM, Frier BM. Oral disorders associated with diabetes mellitus. Diabet Med 1992;9:410-416.
3. Meara JG, Shah S, Li KK, Cunningham MJ. The odontogenic keratocyst: a 20-year clinicopathologic review. Laryngoscope 1998;108:280-283.
4. Williams TP, Connor FA Jr. Surgical management of the odontogenic keratocyst: aggressive approach. J Oral Maxillofac Surg 1994;52:964-966.
5. Meiselman F. Surgical management of the odontogenic keratocyst: conservative approach. J Oral Maxillofac Surg 1994;52:960-963.
6. Stoelinga PJ. Long-term follow-up on keratocysts treated according to a defined protocol. Int J Oral Maxillofac Surg 2001;30:14-25.
7. Cawson RA, Odell EW. Cysts of the Jaw. In: Essentials of Oral Pathology and Oral Medicine. Edinburgh: Churchill Livingstone 1997:97-116.
8. Harvey W, Guat-Chen F, Gordon D et al. Evidence for fibroblasts as the major source of prostacyclin and prostaglandin synthesis in dental cyst in man. Arch Oral Biol 1984;29:223-229.
9. Teronen O, Salo T, Laitinen J et al. Characterization of interstitial collagenases in jaw cyst wall. Eur J Oral Sci 1995;103:141-147.
10. Ward JP, Magar V, Franks SJ, Landini G. A mathematical model of the dynamics of odontogenic cyst growth. Anal Quant Cytol Histol 2004;26:39-46.
11. Speight PM, Barrett AW. Salivary gland tumours. Oral Dis 2002;8:229-240.
12. Bryant SR. The effects of age, jaw site, and bone condition on oral implant outcomes. Int J Prosthodont 1998;11:470-490.
13. Sennerby L, Roos J. Surgical determinants of clinical success of osseointegrated oral implants: a review of the literature. Int J Prosthodont 1998;11:408-420.
14. Esposito M, Hirsch JM, Lekholm U, Thomsen P. Biological factors contributing to failures of osseointegrated oral implants (II). Etiopathogenesis. Eur J Oral Sci 1998;106:721-764.
15. Berne RM, Levy MN, Koeppen BM, Stanton BM. Hormones of the Pancreatic Islets. In: Physiology. London: Mosby 1998:832-840.
16. Harrison JS, Dale RA, Haveman CW, Redding SW. Oral complications in radiation therapy. Gen Dent 2003;51:552-560.
17. Shaw MJ, Kumar ND, Duggal M et al. Oral management of patients following oncology treatment: literature review. Br J Oral Maxillofac Surg 2000;38:519-524.
18. Joyston-Bechal S. Management of oral complications following radiotherapy. Dent Update 1992;19:232-234, 236-238.
19. http://www.nice.org.uk (last visited 24/04/04)
20. Report of a working party convened by the faculty of dental surgery; Current clinical practice and parameters of care: The management of patients with Third molar (syn: wisdom) teeth. http://www.rcseng.ac.uk/dental/fds/pdf/3rdmolar.pdf (last visited 24/04/04)
21. Mason DA. Lingual nerve damage following lower third molar surgery. Int J Oral Maxillofac Surg 1988;17:290-294.
22. Rood JP, Shehab BA. The radiological prediction of inferior alveolar nerve injury during third molar surgery. Br J Oral Maxillofac Surg 1990;28:20-25.

23. Robinson PP. Observations on the recovery of sensation following inferior alveolar nerve injuries. Br J Oral Maxillofac Surg 1988;26:177-189.
24. Rood JP. Lingual split technique. Damage to inferior alveolar and lingual nerves during removal of impacted mandibular third molars. Br Dent J 1983;154:402-403.
25. Middlehurst RJ, Barker GR, Rood JP. Postoperative morbidity with mandibular third molar surgery: a comparison of two techniques. J Oral Maxillofac Surg 1988;46:474-476.
26. Rood JP. Permanent damage to inferior alveolar and lingual nerves during the removal of impacted mandibular third molars. Comparison of two methods of bone removal. Br Dent J 1992; 172:108-110.
27. Haskell R. Medico-legal consequences of extracting lower third molar teeth. Med Prot Soc Ann Report 1986;51-52.
28. Smith KG, Robinson PP. An experimental study of three methods of lingual nerve defect repair. J Oral Maxillofac Surg 1995;53:1052-1062.
29. Cooper DS. Hyperthyroidism. Lancet 2003;362:459-468.
30. Greenwood M, Meechan JG. General medicine and surgery for dental practitioners. Part 6: The endocrine system. Br Dent J 2003;195:129-133.
31. Barber HD. Conservative management of the fractured atrophic edentulous mandible. J Oral Maxillofac Surg 2001;59:789-791.
32. Luhr HG, Reidick T, Merten HA. Results of treatment of fractures of the atrophic edentulous mandible by compression plating: a retrospective evaluation of 84 consecutive cases. J Oral Maxillofac Surg 1996;54:250-254; discussion 254-255.
33. Newman L. The role of autogenous primary rib grafts in treating fractures of the atrophic edentulous mandible. Br J Oral Maxillofac Surg 1995;33:381-386; discussion 386-387.
34. Clerehugh V, Tugnait A. Periodontal diseases in children and adolescents: I. Aetiology and diagnosis. Dent Update 2001;28:222-230, 232.
35. Chapple IL. Periodontal diseases in children and adolescents: classification, aetiology and management. Dent Update 1996;23:210-216.
36. Sciubba JJ. Oral precancer and cancer: etiology, clinical presentation, diagnosis and management. Compend Contin Educ Dent 2000;21:892-898, 900-902.
37. Lopez BC, Hamlyn PJ, Zakrzewska JM. Systematic review of ablative neurosurgical techniques for the treatment of trigeminal neuralgia. Neurosurgery 2004;54:973-982; discussion 982-983.
38. Wahlund K, List T, Larsson B. Treatment of temporomandibular disorders among adolescents: a comparison between occlusal appliance, relaxation training, and brief information. Acta Odontol Scand 2003;61:203-211.
39. Harris M, Feinmann C, Wise M, Treasure F. Temporomandibular joint and orofacial pain: clinical and medicolegal management problems. Br Dent J 1993;174:129-136.
40. Jaiarj N. Drug-induced gingival overgrowth. J Mass Dent Soc 2003;52:16-20.
41. Hyland PL, Traynor PS, Myrillas TT et al. The effects of cyclosporin on the collagenolytic activity of gingival fibroblasts. J Periodontol 2003;74:437-445.
42. Rosenberg M, Phero JC. Regional anesthesia and invasive techniques to manage head and neck pain. Otolaryngol Clin North Am. 2003:1201-1219.
43. Merrison AF, Fuller G. Treatment options for trigeminal neuralgia. BMJ 2003;327:1360-1361.
44. Fisher A, Zakrzewska JM, Patsalos PN. Trigeminal neuralgia: current treatments and future developments. Expert Opin Emerg Drugs 2003;8:123-143.
45. Kodama J, Uchida K, Kushiro H et al. Hereditary angioneurotic edema and thromboembolic diseases: I: How symptoms of acute attacks change with aging. Intern Med 1998;37:440-443.

Bibliography for Part II

Q1.
Feine JS, Carlsson GE. Implant Overdentures. The standard of care for edentulous patients. Surrey: Quintessence Publishing Co. Ltd 2003.
Palmer RM, Smith BJ, Howe LC, Palmer PJ. Implants in clinical dentistry. London: Martin Dunitz 2002.

Q2.
Creugers NH, Kayser AF, Van't Hof MA. A seven-and-a-half-year survival study of resin bonded bridges. J Dent Res 1992;71:1822-1825.
De Kanter RJ, Creugers NH, Verzijden CW, Van't Hof MA. A five year multi-practice clinical study on posterior resin-bonded bridges. J Dent Res 1998;77:609-614.
Djemal S, Setchell D, King P, Wickens J. Long term survival characteristics of 832 resin-retained bridges and splints provided in a post-graduate teaching hospital between 1978 and 1993. J Oral Rehab 1999;26:302-320.
Morgan C, Djemal S, Gilmour, G. Predictable resin bonded bridges in general dental practice. Dent Update 2001;28:501-509.
Wallmsley AD, Walsh TF, Burke TFJ et al. The principles of tooth replacement. In: Restorative Dentistry. London: Churchill Livingstone 2002.

Q3.
Palacci P. Esthetic Implant Dentistry. Soft and hard tissue management. Surrey: Quintessence Publishing Co. Ltd 2001.
Palmer RM, Smith BJ, Howe LC, Palmer PJ. Implants in Clinical Dentistry. London: Martin Dunitz 2002.
Watson CJ, Tinsley D, Sharma S. Implant complications and failures: the single tooth restoration. Dent Update 2000;27:35-43.

Q4.
Magne P, Belser U. Bonded porcelain restorations in the anterior dentition. A biomimetric approach. Surrey: Quintessence Publishing Co. Ltd 2002.
Walls AW, Steele JG, Wassell RW. Crowns and extra coronal restorations: porcelain laminate veneers. Br Dent J 2002;193:73-76.

Q5.
Lim KC. Considerations in intracoronal bleaching. Aust Endod J 2004;30:69-73.

Q6.
Bartlett DW. Bleaching discoloured teeth. Dent Update 2001;28:14-19.
Harrington GW, Natkin E. External resorption associated with bleaching of pulpless teeth. J Endodont 1979;5:344-348.
Lim KC. Considerations in intracoronal bleaching. Aust Endod J 2004;30:69-73.

Q7.
Barker P, Spedding C. The aetiology of gingival recession. Dent Update 2002;29:59-63.

Q8.
Allen PF. Use of tooth coloured restorations in the management of toothwear. Dent Update 2003;30:550-556.
Chu FCS, Siu ASC, Newsome PRH et al. Restorative management of the worn dentition: 2. Localized anterior toothwear. Dent Update 2002;29:214-222.
King P. Restorative management of the worn dentition. In: Addy M, Embery G, Edgar WM, Orchardson R (eds). Tooth Wear and Sensitivity. Clinical advances in restorative dentistry. London: Martin Duntitz 2000.

Q9.
Barker P. The management of gingival recession. Dent Update 2002;29:114-126.

Q10.
Basker RM, DavenPort JL. Prosthetic treatment of the edentulous patient (4th edition). Oxford: Blackwell Munksgaard. 2002:146-171.
Chan MFW-Y, Adams D, Brudvick JS. The swinglock removable partial denture in clinical practice. Dent Update 1998;25:80-84.

Q11.
Chapple ILC, Lumley PJ. The periodontal–endodontic interface. Dent Update 1999;26:331-343.

Q12.
Addy M. The use of antiseptics in periodontal therapy. In: Lindhe J, Karring T, Lang T (eds) Clinical Periodontology and Implants (4th edition). Oxford: Blackwell Munksgaard 2003:464-493.
Watts A, Addy M. Tooth discolouration and staining: a review of the literature. Br Dent J 2001;24:309-316.

Q13.
Basker RM, DavenPort JL. Prosthetic treatment of the edentulous patient (4th edition). Blackwell Munksgaard. 2002:146-171.
McCord JF, Grant AA. Identification of complete denture problems: a summary. Br Dent J 2000;189:128-134.

Q14.
Butterworth C, Chapple I. Drug induced gingival overgrowth: a case with auto-correction of incisor drifting. Dent update 2001;28:411-417.
Camargo PM, Melnick PR, Pirih FQ et al. Treatment of drug induced gingival enlargement: aesthetic and functional considerations. Periodontol 2000 2001;27:131-138.
Scully C, Cawson RA. Medical problems in dentistry (5th edition). Oxford: Churchill Livingston 2005:520-545.

Q15
Berfenholtz G, Hørsted-Bindslev P, Reit C. Text book of endodontology. Oxford: Blackwell Munksguaard 2003.

Bibliography for Part II

Stankiewicz NR, Wilson PR. The ferrule effect: a literature review. Int Endod J 2002;35:575-581.
Stewardson DA. Non-metal post systems. Dent Update 2001;28:326-336.

Q16
Holmstrup P, Westergaard J. Necrotizing periodontal disease. In: Lindhe J, Karring T, Lang T (eds). Clinical Periodontology and Implants (4th edition). Oxford: Blackwell Munksgaard 2003:243-259.
Scully C, Cawson RA. Medical problems in dentistry (5th edition). Oxford: Churchill Livingston 2005:205-230.

Q17.
Lynch CD, McConnell RJ. The use of microabrasion to remove discoloured enamel: a clinical report. J Prosthet Dent 2003;90:417-419.
Welbury RR, Duggal MS, Hosey M-T. Paediatric dentistry. Oxford: Oxford University Press 2005:171-198.

Q18.
Shillingburg Jr HT, Hobo S, Whitseth LD et al. Fundamentals of fixed prosthodontics (3rd edition). Surrey: Quintessence Publishing Co. Ltd 1997.

Q19.
Jenkins G. Precision attachments. A link to successful restorative treatment. Surrey: Quintessence Publishing Co. Ltd 1999.

Q20.
Berfenholtz G, Hørsted-Bindslev P, Reit C. Text book of endodontology. Oxford: Blackwell Munksguaard 2003.

Q21.
British National Formulary. No 51 (Dinesh Mehta, ed). London: BMJ Publishing Group Ltd, March 2006.
Palmer NA. Revisiting the role of prescribing. Dent Update 2003;30:570-574.

Q22.
Davenport JC, Basker RM, Heath JR et al. A clinical guide to removable partial dentures. London: BDJ Books 2000.

Q23.
Packer ME, Davis DM. The long term management of patients with tooth surface loss treated using removable appliances. Dent Update 2000;27:454-459.
Hemmings KW, Howlett JA, Woodley NJ, Griffiths BM. Partial dentures for patients with advanced toothwear. Dent Update 1995;22:52-59.
Toolson LB, Taylor TD. A 10 year report of a longitudinal recall of overdenture patients. J Prosthet Dent 1989;62:179-181.

Q24.
Allen PF. Use of tooth coloured restorations in the management of toothwear. Dent Update. 2003;30:550-556.
Chu FCS, Yip HK, Newsome PRH et al. Restorative management of the worn dentition: aetiology and diagnosis. Dent Update 2002;29:162-169.
Dahl BL, Krogstad OK, Karlsen K. An alternative treatment in cases with localized attrition. J Oral Rehabil 1975;2:209-214.
King P. Restorative management of the worn dentition. In: Addy M, Embery G, Edgar WM, Orchardson R (eds). Tooth Wear and Sensitivity. Clinical advances in restorative dentistry. London: Martin Duntitz 2000.

Q25.
Van Noort R. Introduction to dental materials (2nd edition). London: Mosby 2002.

Index

A

abutments 144
    ball-ended 108
acanthoma 86
Actinobacillus actinomycetemcomitans 66
aesthetics 110, 111-112, 124, 126, 139, 154
albumin 90
alcohol 33, 34, 71, 72, 88
allergy 31
allograft 54
alloplastic material 54
alopecia 78, 101
ameloblastoma 10, 42
amitryptilline 77
amlodipine 38, 68
amoxycillin 64
anaemia 6, 73, 78
    chronic 72
    investigations 101
    pernicious 29
anaesthesia
    caused by axonotmesis 51
    general 26
    inadequate 23
    local 26
    permanent 23
    prolonged 23
Andrew's six keys of occlusion 83
angina 31, 35, 36, 61
angular bone loss 66
antibiotics 4, 26, 49, 63, 64
antibody 69, 70
antigen 69
aphthous ulcers, recurrent 28
arthritis 9, 31, 71
    osteoarthritis 61, 74-76
    rheumatoid 74-76
aspiration 10, 16, 19, 23
aspirin 15, 31, 35, 36, 37, 38, 39, 68, 85, 100
asthma 7, 9, 10, 31, 41, 82, 100
atenolol 15, 28, 35, 38, 68, 85
atheroma 36
atorvastatin 68
atrial fibrillation 74

atrophic 23, 59
    candidiasis 8
    mandible 62
atypical facial pain 78
autoantibodies 29, 48, 59, 70
autogenous bone 46
axonotmesis 51
azathioprine 30

B

bacterial endocarditis 59
bactericidal 64
Bacteroides sp 66
basal cell carcinoma 11, 33, 34
basal cell papilloma 86
basic periodontal examination 32
beclomethasone dipropionate 41, 61, 101
Behçet's disease 29, 30
betamethasone 30, 49
betel nut 34, 72
bifid ribs 11
bimaxillary osteotomy 82
biopsy 10, 13, 73, 94, 101
    gingival 48
    incisional 10, 34
    mucosal 48
bleaching, internal 116, 117-118
bleeding 81
    disorders 22, 23
    features of lesion 34
    freckle 33, 34
    gums 47
    intraoperative 84
    post-extraction 39
    post-operative 85
    retrobulbar 46
    socket 38
blood blisters 68
blow-out fracture 45
bone graft 54, 111-112
bony expansion 93
bullae 101
    intact 69
    intraepithelial 69
    subepithelial 69
bullous lichen planus 69

C

C-Factor 155-156
C1 esterase inhibitor 92
calcification 94
    falx cerebri 11
calcifying epithelial odontogenic tumour (Pindborg tumour) 94
calcium hydroxide 145-146
cancer, oral 102-104 (*see also* malignancy)
candidal
    assessment 8, 29
    imprints 101
    infection 7, 72, 73, 78, 101
    rinses 101
candidosis 72
Capnocytophaga sp 66
carbamazepine 78
carcinoma
    basal cell 33, 34
    malignant 34
    metastatic thyroid 56
    squamous cell 34, 63, 72, 86
    in situ 72
caries 26, 42, 56, 59, 60
    control 103
    extensive root 32
    radiation 104
    subgingival 91
cemental dysplasia 94
cementifying fibroma 94
cementoblastoma 94
chlorhexidine 130, 146
chlorhexidine gluconate 30, 48
cholesterol clefts 89
chronic adult periodontitis 36, 56
chronic bronchitis 88
cicatricial pemphigoid 48, 69
clonidine 100
coagulation factors 92
co-amoxiclav 64
coeliac disease 29
competent lips 83
complement 92
composites 153-154
computerised tomograph (CT) 45
condyles 89, 98
connective tissue disease 59
consent 42, 87, 97, 98
corticosteroids 30, 49, 59

Crohn's disease 29, 133-134
crossbites 83
crowding 83
crowns 116, 136, 144
    preparations 141-142
cryotherapy 78
cyclo-oxygenase 36, 37
cyclosporin 85, 86
cyst 12
    dentigerous 10, 42
    growth 14
    neoplastic 13
    non-odontogenic 13
    odontogenic 13, 42
    periodontal 13
    protein 90
    pseudocysts 13
    radicular 88, 89
    residual 10, 13
    satellite 89
    subchondral 76

D

Dahl concept 153-154
dental lamina 89
dental trauma 21-24, 53-54
Dentatus articulator 22
dentine, bonding 155-157
dento-skeletal relationship 82
dentures 107, 131-132, 143-144, 151-152
    anatomy 131-132
    complex cases 143-144
    designing 149-150
    full upper 32
    overdentures 107, 108, 150, 152
    partial 125-126, 144, 149, 150, 151
    swinglock 126
    toothwear 151-152
depression 7, 77, 81
dermatitis herpetiformis 69
desquamative gingivitis 47
diabetes mellitus 6, 7, 22, 25-27, 67
    control 36
    gestational 26
    poorly controlled 8
    secondary 26
    Type I, insulin-dependent 25-26, 35
    Type II, non-insulin dependent 26

Index

diazepam 85
diet counselling 32
dipyridamole 100
discoloured tooth 115-116, 117, 129-130, 139-140
disseminated intravascular coagulation (DIC) 91, 92
DNA synthesis 64
Down syndrome 67
doxazocin 77
doxycycline 49
dry mouth 16, 58-59, 95, 96
dysplasia 72, 73
    cemental 94

E

eczema 47, 100
edentulous
    jaw 107
    mandible 108
    maxilla 108, 151
    ridges 131-132
Ehlers Danlos syndrome, Type VIII 67
Eikenella corrodens 66
emphysema 61
endocarditis, infective 147-148
endodontic
    irrigants 145
    treatment 128, 146
enophthalmos 45
Enterococcus faecalis 146
enucleation 10, 94
eosinophilic granuloma 67
epidermolysis bullosa 69
epilepsy 18, 74
epithelial rests of malassez 89
erosions
    healing 69
    multiple 8, 69
    periarticular 76
    white patch 101
erosive lichen planus 8, 100
erythema 48, 72, 101
    multiforme 69
erythroplakia 72
extirpation 54
extraction 26, 32, 36, 39, 54, 62, 64, 94

F

5-nitroimidazole 64
facial
    deformity 82-84
    laceration 79-81
    nerve 15, 17, 20
    course 80
    weakness 80
    pain 77-78
    trauma 97-99
ferrule 136
fibre posts 135-136
    glass-fibre posts 135
fibrinolysis 92
fibroblast proliferation 86
fibroepithelial polyp 86, 96
fixed bridges 107, 108
fluoride 31, 32, 36, 59, 103
fluorosis 139-140
folate 8, 29, 78
formol-saline 34, 42, 87
fracture, of mandible 62, 98
freckle 33, 34
free end saddles 125-126
frictional keratosis 72
frontal bossing 11
frusemide 68, 77, 85

G

gabapentin 100
genetic syndromes 67
gingiva 47, 48, 83, 104, 137
gingival
    disease 137-138
    enlargement 133-134
    fibromatosis, hereditary 134
    hyperplasia 85, 86, 134
    margin 69, 114
    recession 119-120, 123-124, 126
    tissue 112
gingivitis 47, 48, 83
    necrotic ulcerative 137-138
glass ionomer cement 32
glossitis 8
glycerol trinitrate (GTN) 68
glyceryl trinitrate 31, 38
gold bar 108
Gorlin Goltz syndrome 11
gram-negative bacteria 64

gram-positive bacteria 64
grinding 74
gums, painful 47-49, 137-138

H

haemorrhage 23, 43, 92
haemosiderin 89
haemostasis 39
hereditary angioedema 91-92
herpes zoster 69
Herztel exophthalmometry 45
Hess chart 45, 46
HIV infection 67, 96, 138
hormones 29, 48
human bites 3-6
hyperbaric oxygen 64
hypertension 9, 10, 31, 38, 39
hyperglycaemia 26
hypocellularity 103
hypoglycaemia 26
hypophosphatasia 67
hypovascularity 103
hypoxia 103

I

ibuprofen 71
Ig 90
IgG autoantibody 69, 70
immune complexes 59
immunodeficiencies 67
immunofluorescence
    direct 48, 69-70
    indirect 48, 70
immunosupression 133-134
implants 21, 22, 57, 60, 107-108, 111-112
    aesthetics 111-112
    edentulous patient 107-108
    fixed bridges 107-108
    overdentures 107-108
    surgery, complications 23
infection 6, 8, 23, 26, 27, 32, 36, 42, 43, 53, 56, 59, 61, 62, 64, 66, 67, 72, 73, 78, 81, 84, 96, 98, 101
infective endocarditis 147-148
inferior dental nerve, injury 50
internal resorption 54
internal bleaching 116, 117-118

intracranial
    hypertension 148
    tumour 78
ipratropium bromide 61
iron 8, 29, 78

K

keratinised epithelium
    ortho 89
    para 89
keratinocyte growth factor 86

L

lamina dura 13, 89
lamina propria 69
laminate veneers 113-114
lansoprazole 41, 68
leukopenia 67
leukoplakia 71-72
Libman-Sacks vegetations 59
lichen planus 29, 48, 59, 69, 72, 101
    erosive 8, 100
lichenoid reactions 8, 48
lip
    lesion 33-34, 86
    lump 85-86
lipolysis 27
lisinopril 15, 38, 85
localised aggressive periodontitis (LAP) 66
lower face height 83
lupus erythematosus 8, 48, 58, 59, 72
lymphadenopathy 15, 16, 34, 93

M

magnets 108
malignancy
    assessing risk 73
    histological features 34
    hyperproteinaemia 6
    melanoma 33, 34
    oral 102-104
mandibular
    fractures 10, 62, 98
    radiolucency 50-52, 88-90
marsupialisation 10
masseter 80
mattress suture 39
maxillary antrum 45

Index

medical history 4, 7, 15, 16, 17, 29, 35, 36, 38, 39, 41, 58, 61, 62, 87, 100
menopause 48
metabolic acidosis 27
metal posts 135-136
metronidazole 64
microabrasion 140
microneurosurgery 51
microvascular decompression 78
mouth, sore 68-70
MRI scan 78, 86
myocardial infarct 38

N

nabumetone 100
naevoid basal cell carcinoma 11
nasolabial angle 83
neck dissection 86, 103
necrotic ulcerative gingivitis (NUG) 138
neuropraxia 51
neurotmesis 51
NICE guidelines 42
Non-keratinised stratified squamous epithelium 89
Non-vital bleaching 117-118
NSAIDs 59, 101

O

odontogenic fibroma 94
odontogenic keratocyst 9, 10, 11, 13, 42, 50, 52, 88, 89
oedema 6, 92
open reduction and internal fixation 62, 98
oral hygiene 22, 26, 31, 32, 36, 48, 56, 57, 66, 86, 103
orbit
    anatomy 45
    fracture 45, 46
orthodontic 65, 66, 82, 83
orthognathic surgery, complications 84
osseointegration 21, 24, 53, 54, 108
    mandible 108
    maxilla 108
osteoarthritis 61, 74-76
    Bouchard's nodes 75
    Heberden's nodes 75
    joint deformities 75
    X-ray changes 76

osteomyelitis 64
osteoradionecrosis 64, 103
overdentures 107, 108, 144, 152

P

pain 31-32, 55-57, 91-92
palatal toothwear 121-122
palmor pitting 11
papilloma 86, 96
Papillon-Lefèvre syndrome 67
parotid gland
    anatomy 17, 80
    lipoma 16
    lump investigation 16
    swelling 15-17
    tumour
        benign 17
        malignant 17
partial denture 12, 32, 36, 57, 58, 59, 125-126, 144, 149-150, 151
patch-testing 48
pathological fracture of mandible 62
pemphigoid 48, 49
pemphigus 48
    vegetans 69
    vulgaris 69
penicillin
    allergy to 30, 82
    broad-spectrum 64
    exacerbating SLE 59
peptic ulceration 41
periapical
    abscess 39, 54, 56, 92
    granuloma 56
    infection 56
    intraoral 53
    periodontitis 92
    pathology 42
    radiographs 32, 54, 65, 66
    radiolucency 36, 54
    widening 26
periodontal
    abscess 36, 39
    splints 119-120
perio-endo lesion 39, 127-128
pernicious anaemia 29
Pindborg tumour 94
plaque 32, 69, 83, 86
plasma, fresh frozen 92

169

platelets 37, 92
    aggregation 36
pleomorphic adenoma 17, 18
    histology 19
polyuria 8, 27
precision attachments 143-144
prednisolone 49, 61, 85
preorthognathic decompensation 83
proptosis 45
prostacyclin 36, 37
protein
    analysis 10
    breakdown 27
    measurement 89
    nutritional deficiency 6
    serum 90
    soluble 10, 90
    stores 27
protozoa 64
psoriasis 48
psychogenic facial pain 78
pulpitis, irreversible 32, 56

R

radial forearm microvascular free flap 63, 103
radiolucency
    apical 56
    mandible 9, 10, 12-14, 50
    multilocular 51
    periapical 36, 54
    right mental foramen region 13
    unerupted lower right 10, 42
    unilocular 42
radio-opacity 93-94
radiotherapy 6, 64, 96, 102
    effects
        bone 103
        mucosa 104
        teeth 104
    post-operative 63
ramipril 68
ranitidine 85
recession 56
    gingival 48, 119-120, 123-124, 126
renal transplant 85
resin-retained bridge 22, 109-110
    advantages over conventional bridge 110

resin-retained bridge
    disadvantages over conventional bridge 110
    fixed-fixed, reasons for failure 110
    lower success rate 110
resistance 142
retention 142, 144, 150
rheumatoid arthritis 74-76
    joint swelling 75
    swan neck/boutonniere deformities 75
    ulnar deviation 75
    X-ray changes 76
rib-grafting 62
root
    canal therapy (RCT) 64
        treatment 145-146
    caries 32, 36
    facial motor 80
    filling 53, 89
    fractured 22, 43
    infected 61, 62
    mesial 51
    planing 57 66
    resorption 89
    retained 61-62

S

salbutamol 31, 41
salicylate 30
saliva substitute 59
sarcoidosis 48
scaling 32, 36, 56, 57, 66, 86, 103
scars 69
silastic sheet 46
sinus 16, 19, 23, 53, 54, 63-64, 93
Sjögren's syndrome 8
Skeletal pattern, Class II 83
smoking 72, 82, 86
sore gums 47-49
sore mouth 68-70
sore tongue 7-8
squamous cell carcinoma 34, 63, 72
    lip 86
stress 26, 29, 60, 81, 92
striations 8, 69
stroke 74
sublingual space 61, 62

Index

submandibular gland 18
    anatomy 19
    examination 19
    investigation 19
    surgery 20
        anatomy 20
        complications 20
    swelling 18-20
sulphonamides 59
supragingival scaling 36, 56
surgery
    factors influencing success 124
    second stage 111
surgical excision 73, 86
surveying 150
suturing (skin) 4
swab 8, 29, 64
swinglock denture 126
systemic lupus erythematosus 8, 48, 58, 59

T

temporomandibular joint (TMJ) 78, 89
    clicking 74
    deviation on opening 74
    disorders 74-76
        temporomandibular joint dysfunction syndrome (TMJD) 75
        management TMJD 75
    limitation opening 74
    pain 74
    tenderness 74
tetracycline 66, 101
    mouthwash 30
third molar surgery 42
    complications 43
thromboxane A2 36
thyrotoxicosis 55, 61
    causes 56
    clinical features 56
titanium
    fracture plates 46, 98
    mesh 46
TMJ *see* temporomandibular joint
tongue 8, 72
    burning 77, 78
    lesion on dorsum 96
    loss of motor supply 20
    loss of sensation and taste 20
    lump 95-96

tongue
    sore 7-8
    white patch 71
toothache 35-37
toothwear
    composites 153-154
    dentures 151-152
    palatal 121-122
torque testing 54
treatment planning 21
triamcinolone 30, 101
trigeminal ganglion 78
trigeminal neuralgia 78
tuberculosis 29

U

ulcers 8, 28, 29
    hard palate 8
    lips 100
    mucosa 29
    multiple intraoral 29
    oral 28-30, 100-101
unerupted third molar 42, 98

V

veneers 113-114, 116, 121-122
verapamil 31
vesiculobullous disease 29
vitality tests 13, 32, 57
vitamin B12 8, 29

W

white patch 69, 71-73, 101
white striae 59, 101
Wickham's striae 101
wire 64
wound healing 3-6, 27
    impaired 6
    phases
        inflammatory phase 5
        proliferative phase 5
        remodelling phase 5

X

xenograft 54
xerostomia 8, 58-59, 95, 96, 104

Z

zinc chloride 30